STUDY GUIDE

Patty Rosenberger
Cori Ann Ramírez

Colorado State University

ABNORMAL PSYCHOLOGY IN A CHANGING WORLD

THIRD EDITION

Jeffrey S. Nevid

Spencer A. Rathus

Beverly Greene

St. John's University

PRENTICE HALL, *Upper Saddle River, New Jersey 07458*

© 1997 by PRENTICE-HALL, INC.
Simon & Schuster / A Viacom Company
Upper Saddle River, New Jersey 07458

10 9 8 7 6 5 4 3 2 1

ISBN 0-13- 552655-8
Printed in the United States of America

TABLE OF CONTENTS

PREFACE

Your textbook is a comprehensive review of the fascinating area of abnormal psychology, emphasizing the most recent clinical knowledge while describing the types of research methods used in this field. This study guide has been developed to complement your textbook and facilitate your understanding the material that is presented in each chapter.

The following study guide follows your text on a chapter by chapter basis. There are several sections that are arranged to help you thoroughly review the material in the text. First, an **OVERVIEW** briefly summarizes the central purposes of the chapter. This is followed by a **CHAPTER OUTLINE** which will provide a roadmap of what you will be reading. The chapter **LEARNING OBJECTIVES** printed in your text are reprinted in this study guide for your convenience. The next section features **KEY TERMS AND CONCEPTS** that are important for you to understand. This is followed by **MATCHING, TRUE-FALSE**, and **MULTIPLE CHOICE** sections, which are designed to facilitate integrating the information presented in the text. Answers to these sections are found at the end of each study guide chapter. Finally, each lesson ends by posing some **QUESTIONS FOR CRITICAL THINKING** that are drawn from discussions in the text on important topics.

We hope that this study guide will be a valuable resource for you this semester as you review the material presented in your textbook. Reading through the sections carefully and completing all of the exercises should prove to be helpful as you prepare for exams. Good luck in your course!

CHAPTER ONE

WHAT IS ABNORMAL PSYCHOLOGY?

OVERVIEW

This chapter introduces the field of abnormal psychology; it is divided into four major sections. The first defines and illustrates the concept of abnormal behavior. The second considers cultural biases.

The third major section traces the history of abnormal behavior. You will quickly come to appreciate that the way society viewed abnormal behavior was a major determinant of how society treated mental illness. This is still true today. Contemporary psychologists have developed several different models of abnormal behavior, and the third section ends with an introduction to six major viewpoints.

The final section explores research methods used in abnormal psychology. Much of our knowledge of abnormal behavior is the result of application of scientific method. This section provides a brief review of scientific method and then elaborates on specific research methods that are widely used to study abnormal behavior and its treatment.

CHAPTER OUTLINE

What is Abnormal Behavior?
Cultural Bases of Abnormal Behavior
Historical Perspectives on Abnormal Behavior
    The Demonological Model
    Origins of the Medical Model: In "Ill Humor"
    Medieval Times
    Witchcraft
        Asylums
    The Rise of Modern Thought
        Advances in Medicine
        Emil Kraepelin
    The Reform Movement and Moral Therapy
        A Step Backward
        The Contemporary Exodus from State Hospitals
    Pathways to the Present
        Psychodynamic Perspectives
        Learning Perspectives
        Humanistic-Existential Perspectives
        Cognitive Perspectives
        Sociocultural Perspectives
        Eclectic Models

Research Methods in Abnormal Psychology
    Description, Explanation, Prediction, and Control: The Objectives of
Science
        The Scientific Method
        The Naturalistic-Observation Method
        Correlation
        The Longitudinal Study
        The Experimental Method
                Experimental and Control Subjects
                Random Assignment
                Controlling for Subjects' Expectations
                Placebo-Control Studies
                Experimental Validity
                    Analogue Studies
        Quasi-Experimental Methods
        Epidemiological Method
        The Case-Study Method
                Types of Case Studies
                The Single-Case Experimental Design
Summary

LEARNING OBJECTIVES

The following learning objectives can also be found at the beginning of the chapter.
When you have completed your study of the chapter, you should be able to:

1.   Discuss six criteria used to define abnormal behavior.
2.   Discuss the relationships between cultural beliefs and norms and the
      labeling of behavior as normal or abnormal.
3.   Recount the history of the demonological approach to abnormal behavior,
      referring to ancient and medieval times.
4.   Describe the contributions of Hippocrates, Galen, Weyer, Pasteur,
      Griesinger, and Kraepelin to the development of medical science and
      thinking.
5.   Describe the development of treatment centers for abnormal behavior from
      asylums through the mental hospital.
6.   Discuss the reform movement and the use of moral therapy, focusing on
      the roles of Pussin, Pinel, Rush, and Dix.
7.   Discuss the factors associated with the current exodus from mental
      hospitals in the United States.
8.   Discuss various contemporary concepts or models of abnormal behavior.
9.   Discuss the objectives of a scientific approach to the study of abnormal
      behavior.
10.   Describe the steps involved in the scientific method.

11. Discuss the value and limitations of the naturalistic-observation method.
12. Discuss the importance of drawing representative samples from target populations.
13. Discuss the value and limitations of correlational research.
14. Discuss longitudinal research.
15. Describe the purpose and features of the experimental method.
16. Explain ways in which experimenters control for subjects' and researchers' expectations.
17. Describe three types of experimental validity.
18. Discuss the value of, and sources of error in, the epidemiological method.
19. Discuss the value and limitations of the case-study method.
20. Provide examples of single-case experimental designs and explain how they help researchers.

KEY TERMS AND CONCEPTS

The following is a list of terms, concepts, and names that are discussed in the chapter. They are important for you to know. Review these terms, comparing your answers with the material presented in the text.

Abnormal psychology
Medical model
Hallucinations
Delusions
Agoraphobic
Schizophrenia
Models
Comorbidity
Demonology
Possession
Trephining
Demonological Model
Hippocrates
Humors
Phlegmatic
Melancholia
Sanguine
Choleric
Galen
Exorcism
Johann Weyer
Asylums
Edward Jenner
Louis Pasteur

Joseph Lister
Gregor Mendel
Robert Koch
Wilhelm Griesinger
Emil Kraepelin
Demential praecox
Bipolar disorder
General paresis
Jean-Baptiste Pussin
Philippe Pinel
Moral Therapy
William Tuke
Dorothea Dix
Benjamin Rush
Phenothiazines
Deinstitutionalization
Jean-Martin Charcot
Joseph Breuer
Sigmund Freud
Friedrich Mesmer
Mesmerism
Hypnosis
Anna O
Catharsis
Psychoanalytic theory
Psychodynamic model
Free association
Ivan Pavlov
John B. Watson
Behaviorism
B.F. Skinner
Behavior therapy
Social-learning theory
Carl Rogers
Abraham Maslow
Existentialism
Martin Heidegger
Jean-Paul Sartre
Self-actualization
Phenomenological perspective
Albert Ellis
Aaron Beck
Cognitive behavior therapy
Eclectic
Inference

Theories
Scientific method
Hypothesis
Antisocial personality disorder
Significant difference
Naturalistic-observation method
Correlation
Variables
Positive correlation
Negative correlation
Longitudinal study
Causal relationship
Experimental method
Independent variables
Dependent variables
Experimental subjects
Control subjects
Selection factor
Blind study
Placebo
Single-blind placebo-control study
Internal validity
External validity
Random sample
Analogue study
In vivo
Construct validity
Quasi-experiments
Obsessive-compulsive disorder
Epidemiological method
Survey method
Incidence
Prevalence
Sample
Random sample
Stratified random sample
Case study
Single case experimental designs
Reversal design
Multiple-baseline design
Modeling
Feedback

MATCHING

Match the following names, terms, and concepts with the definitions listed below. The answers are found at the end of the chapter.

a. naturalistic observation
b. comorbidity
c. deinstitutionalization
d. exorcism
e. Dorothea Dix
f. independent variable
g. causal relationships
h. abnormal psychology
i. longitudinal research
j. eclectic model
k. moral therapy
l. quasi-experiment
m. behavior therapy

n. John B. Watson
o. psychodynamic theory
p. Benjamin Rush
q. medical model
r. case study
s. double-blind
t. scientific method
u. random assignment
v. trephining
w. correlation
x. asylums
y. epidemiological method
z. sociocultural theory

1) _____ studies the description, causes, and treatment of abnormal behavior

2) _____ early institutions for housing mentally ill

3) _____ believed madness was caused by engorgement of blood vessels

4) _____ trend resulting from the Community Mental Health Centers Act and tranquilizers

5) _____ crusader whose efforts led to the establishment of 32 mental hospitals in the USA

6) _____ abnormal behavior explained by an underlying biological or biochemical disorder

7) _____ combines views of multiple models to explain abnormal behavior

8) _____ the perspective that abnormal behavior is caused by stress resulting from poverty and lack of opportunity

9) _____ the perspective the abnormal behavior is the result of unconscious psychological conflicts

10) _____ the process of formulating a question, developing and testing a hypothesis, and drawing conclusions

11) _____ unobtrusively observing behavior as it happens in the natural environment

12) _____ the study of the same subjects over a long period of time

13) _____ manipulated by the scientist, this is the "cause" in a cause-effect relationship

14) _____ an experimental method that lacks random assignment

15) _____ concerned with incidence of abnormal behavior in different population groups but not with specific cause-effect relationships

16) _____ rich in clinical material but lacking in scientific rigor

17) _____ the perspective that normal behavior can be restored by providing humane treatment in a relaxed, positive environment

18) _____ the application of learning principles to overcome psychological problems

19) _____ two events in sequence where the first determines the second

20) _____ a research design that controls for subject and experimenter expectancy effects

21) _____ eliminates the selection factor as an explanation for experimental results

22) _____ refers to the co-occurrence of two or more disorders

23) _____ a harsh method of creating a pathway through the skull to provide an outlet for irascible spirits

24) _____ a treatment for abnormal behavior, this was employed to persuade evil spirits that the bodies of their intended victims were basically uninhabitable

25) _____ the father of behaviorism

26) _____ a statistical measure of the relationships between two factors

TRUE-FALSE

The following true-false statements are reprinted here from your text. Can you remember the answers? They can be found at the end of this chapter.

1. _____ Abnormal behavior affects virtually everyone.
2. _____ Unusual behavior is by definition abnormal.
3. _____ Behavior that is normal in one culture may be regarded as abnormal in another.
4. _____ Many Native Americans claim to hear the spirits of people who have recently died calling to them as they ascend to the afterlife.
5. _____ Innocent people were drowned in medieval times as a way of certifying they were not possessed by the devil.
6. _____ An 18th-century physician discovered that imbalances in magnetic fluids in the body could cause psychological problems such as hysteria.
7. _____ Native Hawaiians lead a carefree existence.
8. _____ In order to carry out valid research, it may be necessary to keep people unaware of the treatments they receive.
9. _____ Case studies have been conducted on people who have been dead for hundreds of years.

MULTIPLE CHOICE

The multiple choice questions listed below will test your understanding of the material presented in the chapter. Read through each question and circle the letter representing the best answer. The answers are found at the end of the chapter.

1) Persistent alcohol use may be labeled abnormal primarily because it:

    a. is statistically uncommon
    b. is maladaptive or self-defeating
    c. is dangerous to others
    d. violates social norms

2) Researchers in Los Angeles found that psychiatric diagnoses:

    a. were virtually identical in various ethnic groups
    b. differed across ethnic groups
    c. were absent in ethnic minorities
    d. were always more common in whites that in other groups

3) Which of the following is NOT consistent with the demonological model?

   a. exorcism
   b. persecution of mentally ill as witches
   c. excessive black bile as the cause of depression
   d. sending patients to temples dedicated to Asclepius, and providing
      nutrition and exercise

4) Which of the following is TRUE of naturalistic observation?

   a. it provides considerable information about behavior but cannot
      specify why a behavior occurs
   b. it is conducted through quasi-experiments
   c. it frequently employs surveys
   d. it is of little value for studying abnormal behavior

5) According to Hippocrates, depression was caused by:

   a. phlegm
   b. yellow bile
   c. blood
   d. black bile

6) Benjamin Rush, the father of American psychiatry, advanced the moral therapy
movement by:

   a. encouraging staff at his Philadelphia Hospital to treat patients with
      kindness and understanding
   b. signing the Patients Human Rights Bill
   c. freeing mental patients from their chains
   d. crusading across the USA against deplorable conditions in jails and
      almshouses

7) A research method that is costly and requires a time commitment that may outlive
the original scientists is called a(n):

   a. longitudinal study
   b. analogue study
   c. survey study
   d. epidemiological study

8) Which of the following is a contemporary model of abnormal behavior that emphasizes the need for therapists to learn to view the world from the client's perspective?

a. medical model
b. social learning perspective
c. humanistic-existential perspective
d. psychodynamic perspective

9) Which of the following attempts to explain abnormal behavior in terms of supernatural or divine causes?

a. medical model
b. disease model
c. medieval model
d. demonological model

10) Psychodynamic perspectives see the cause of abnormal behavior in:

a. principles of learning
b. physical disease
c. underlying psychic forces
d. distorted thinking

11) Freud's study of Anna O. was a famous:

a. single-subject experiment
b. single-blind study
c. double-blind study
d. case study

12) Which of the following is NOT an objective of the scientific approach to abnormal behavior?

a. description
b. explanation
c. statistical analysis
d. control

13) The statement "high levels of exercise will induce anorexia nervosa" is an example of a:

    a. research question
    b. hypothesis
    c. test of a hypothesis
    d. conclusion about a hypothesis

14) Which of the following individuals advanced the medical model of abnormal behavior by postulating that dementia praecox and manic-depressive psychosis were due to physical problems?

    a. Emil Kraepelin
    b. Galen
    c. Aaron Beck
    d. Sigmund Freud

15) It is necessary that a research sample be representative of the _____ of interest.

    a. population
    b. experiment
    c. topic
    d. behavior

16) A research study found that the higher someone's intelligence the less likely it is that they will drop out of school. This finding is a:

    a. positive correlation
    b. test of a hypothesis
    c. causal relationship
    d. negative correlation

17) Which of the following is least associated with the current exodus from mental hospitals?

    a. development of major tranquilizers
    b. overcrowding of mental hospitals in the first half of this century
    c. the Community Mental Health Centers Act of 1963
    d. widespread adoption of the medical model of abnormal behavior

18) An experiment is designed to study the effect of level of anxiety on test performance. Test performance is:

    a. determined by random assignment
    b. the independent variable
    c. dependent variable
    d. a self-report measure

19) The extent to which treatment effects can be accounted for by the theoretical mechanisms that are present in the independent variable is called:

    a. construct validity
    b. external validity
    c. internal validity
    d. significance

20) A research method to determine causal relationships when random assignment is not possible is called a:

    a. longitudinal study
    b. quasi-experiment
    c. correlational study
    d. single-blind experiment

21) Mesmerism and hypnosis were early tools of which view?

    a. eclectic
    b. psychoanalytic
    c. sociocultural
    d. humanistic

22) A single-subject research method in the form of A-B-A-B is called:

    a. a longitudinal study
    b. a case study
    c. a multiple-baseline design
    d. a reversal design

23) All of the following were originally associated with psychodynamic perspective EXCEPT:

    a. Joseph Breuer
    b. Ivan Pavlov
    c. Sigmund Freud
    d. Friedrich Mesmer

24) Multiple baseline design does not require which of the following?

    a. baseline phase
    b. treatment phase
    c. reversal phase
    d. research phase

25) All of the following are steps used in the scientific method when testing theoretical assumptions EXCEPT:

    a. formulating a research question
    b. framing the research question in the form of a hypothesis
    c. testing the hypothesis
    d. drawing direct causal relationships about the hypothesis

26) All of the following are true of longitudinal research EXCEPT:

    a. it is time consuming
    b. the results it produces are questionable due to the length of time involved in the study
    c. it is costly
    d. it is relatively uncommon

27) Most commonly reported disorders are:

    a. depression and alcohol dependence
    b. depression and schizophrenia
    c. antisocial personality disorder and alcohol dependence
    d. social phobia and depression

28) Studies show that while anxiety and depression are more common among women, _____ is more common among men.

    a. obsessive compulsive disorder
    b. social phobia
    c. alcohol and substance abuse problems
    d. schizophrenia

29) Which model sees abnormal behavior as clusters of symptoms called syndromes?

    a. medical model
    b. social learning model
    c. behavioral model
    d. humanistic model

30) The first part of a reversal design is called:

    a. baseline
    b. treatment
    c. treatment withdrawal
    d. treatment reinstatement

QUESTIONS FOR CRITICAL THINKING

1. What are examples of behaviors that are considered abnormal in Western culture but are common in some other cultures?
2. Why might ethnic groups differ in their rates of psychiatric diagnoses?
3. How were demonological views translated into treatment strategies?
4. Identify the contributions of Hippocrates and how these contributions continue to be manifested in the field of psychology.
5. Describe what early asylums were like.
6. Discuss why the late 19th century was a step backward for the treatment of mental illness.
7. Identify the arguments for and against deinstitutionalization. Where do you stand on this issue?
8. Discuss the influence of the medical model. Where do you think the field of psychology might be today without the influence of this model?
9. Compare and contrast the perspectives of psychodynamic, humanistic-existential, cognitive, sociocultural, and learning theory. Which are you most comfortable with and why?
10. What is the concept of controlling human behavior and why is it controversial?
11. Discuss why correlation cannot confirm causation.
12. Identify the advantages and disadvantages of longitudinal research.
13. Discuss some of the limitations inherent in case studies.
14. Discuss some of the reasons why single case designs are weak in external validity.
15. Discuss some of the advantages of multiple baseline designs.
16. Discuss how an individual diagnosed with schizophrenia may be treated today. How does this differ with how this same individual may have been treated in the late 15th through the late 17th centuries?

ANSWERS FOR MATCHING

1.	h	10.	t	19.	g
2.	x	11.	a	20.	s
3.	p	12.	i	21.	u
4.	c	13.	f	22.	b
5.	e	14.	l	23.	v
6.	q	15.	y	24.	d
7.	j	16.	r	25.	n
8.	z	17.	k	26.	w
9.	o	18.	m		

TRUE-FALSE ANSWERS

1.	T	4.	T	7.	F
2.	F	5.	T	8.	T
3.	T	6.	T	9.	T

MULTIPLE CHOICE ANSWERS

1.	b	11.	d	21.	b
2.	b	12.	c	22.	d
3.	c	13.	b	23.	b
4.	a	14.	a	24.	c
5.	d	15.	d	25.	d
6.	a	16.	a	26.	b
7.	a	17.	d	27.	a
8.	c	18.	c	28.	c
9.	d	19.	a	29.	a
10.	c	20.	b	30.	a

CHAPTER TWO

THEORETICAL PERSPECTIVES

OVERVIEW

This chapter is organized around six contemporary perspectives. Each perspective is explained in detail, and then critically evaluated in terms of its strengths and weaknesses. Material in this chapter generally correspond to the major sections of the chapter in your text.

The psychodynamic perspective focuses on unconscious, internal psychological conflict as the critical determinant of abnormal behavior. The learning perspective contrasts sharply with this view. Much of the focus of the learning perspective is on factors external to the individual as determinants of behavior. These are the factors that influence learning processes. Cognitive perspectives focus on the role of cognitions, mental processes including perception, memory, thoughts, and problem solving as determinants of abnormal behavior. The humanistic-existential perspective places considerable emphasis on personal freedom and choices we make in the quest for purpose and meaning in our lives. Finally, the sociocultural perspective focuses on social and cultural factors as explanations for abnormal behavior.

The brevity of this section reflects the scope of this area, but not its impact on abnormal psychology. The final perspective that your chapter explores is the biological perspective, which focuses on abnormal behavior with known biological determinants. A focused review of the major concepts of behavioral neural science provides key background information for understanding the representations of these disorders in later chapters.

CHAPTER OUTLINE

Psychodynamic Perspectives
    Sigmund Freud's Theory of Psychosexual Development
        Conscious, Preconscious, Unconscious: The Geography of the Mind
        The Structure of Personality
        Defense Mechanisms
        Stages of Psychosexual Development
    Other Psychodynamic Theorists
    Psychodynamic Perspectives on Normality and Abnormality
        The Continuum of Normality, Neurosis, and Psychosis
        The Abilities to Love and to Work
        Differentiation of the Self
        Compensation for Feelings of Inferiority
        Erikson's Positive Outcomes
    Evaluating Psychodynamic Perspectives
Learning Perspectives

Evaluating Biological Perspectives

Summary

LEARNING OBJECTIVES

The following learning objectives can also be found at the beginning of the chapter. When you have completed your study of the chapter, you should be able to:

1. Describe the basic tenets of Freud's psychodynamic theory.
2. Describe more recent psychodynamic theories, comparing and contrasting them to Freud's views.
3. Critically evaluate psychodynamic theories.
4. Describe behaviorism and the principles of conditioning.
5. Describe social-learning theory and the situation and person variables that influence behavior.
6. Critically evaluate learning theories.
7. Discuss the information-processing approach, and the theoretical contributions of cognitive theorists Albert Ellis and Aaron Beck.
8. Critically evaluate cognitive theories.
9. Outline some tenets of humanistic and existential philosophies.
10. Describe the views of Maslow and Rogers.
11. Critically evaluate humanistic-existential theories.
12. Describe and evaluate sociocultural approaches toward understanding abnormal behavior.
13. Discuss the connections between acculturation and adjustment among immigrant populations.
14. Describe the structure and functions of the nervous system and explain how neurons communicate with each other.
15. Describe the structures of the brain and their functions.
16. Describe the functions of the endocrine system and explain how hormones are implicated in human behavior.
17. Explain how various kinds of studies suggest roles for genetics in abnormal behavior.
18. Critically evaluate theories concerning the relationships between biological structures and processes and abnormal behavior.

KEY TERMS AND CONCEPTS

The following is a list of terms, concepts, and names that are discussed in the chapter. They are important for you to know. Review these terms, comparing your answers with the material presented in the text.

Etiologies

Psychic determinism
Sigmund Freud
Conscious
Preconscious
Unconscious
Defense mechanisms
Repression
Structural hypothesis
Psychic structures
Id
Pleasure principle
Primary process thinking
Ego
Reality principle
Secondary process thinking
Superego
Identification
Moral principle
Ego ideal
Regression
Rationalization
Displacement
Projection
Reaction formation
Denial
Sublimation
Psychoanalysis
Free association
Self-insight
Eros
Libido
Erogenous zones
Psychosexual
Oral stage
Anal stage
Anal fixation
Anal-retentive
Anal-expulsive
Phallic stage
Oedipus complex
Electra complex
Castration anxiety
Latency stage
Genital stage
Pregenital fixations

Carl Jung
Analytical psychology
Collective unconscious
Archetypes
Alfred Adler
Inferiority complex
Creative self
Individual psychology
Neo-Freudians
Karen Horney
Harry Stack Sullivan
Heinz Hartmann
Ego psychology
Erik Erikson
Psychosocial
Ego identity
Role diffusion
Object-relations theory
Margaret Mahler
Neuroses
Phobia
Neurotic anxiety
Reality anxiety
Psychosis
Sir Karl Popper
John B. Watson
Behaviorist movement
B.F. Skinner
Classical conditioning
Ivan Pavlov
Unconditioned stimulus
Unconditioned response
Conditioned stimulus
Conditioned response
"Little Albert"
Extinguish
Spontaneous recovery
Operant conditioning
Reinforcement
Reward
Positive reinforcers
Negative reinforcers
Primary reinforcers
Secondary reinforcers
Punishment

Social-learning theory
Albert Bandura
Julian B. Rotter
Walter Mischel
Person variables
Expectancies
Subjective values
Modeling
Situation variables
Competencies
Encoding
Self-efficacy expectations
Cognition
Albert Ellis
Aaron Beck
Rational emotive therapy
Cognitive therapy
Cognitive distortions
"A-B-C approach"
Catastrophize
Selective abstraction
Overgeneralization
Magnification
Absolutist thinking
Jean-Paul Sartre
Martin Heidegger
Ludwig Binswanger
Medard Boss
Viktor Frankl
Abraham Maslow
Self-actualization
Hierarchy of needs
Carl Rogers
Self theory
Frames of reference
Self-esteem
Unconditional positive regard
Conditional positive regard
Conditions of worth
Person-centered therapy
Self-ideals
Sociocultural perspective
Sociocultural theory
Thomas Szasz
R.D. Laing

Downward drift hypothesis
Acculturation
Melting pot theory
Bicultural theory
Neurons
Soma
Dendrites
Axon
Terminals
Knobs
Neurotransmitters
Synapse
Receptor site
Acetylcholine
Dopamine
Norepinephrine
Epinephrine
Serotonin
Central nervous system
Peripheral nervous system
Medulla
Pons
Cerebellum
Reticular activating system
Comatose
Thalamus
Hypothalamus
Limbic system
Basal ganglia
Cerebrum
Cerebral cortex
Corpos callosum
Somatic nervous system
Autonomic nervous system
Sympathetic nervous system
Parasympathetic nervous system
Endocrine system
Hormones
Steroids
Corticosteroids
Hypoglycemia
Thyroxin
Cretinism
Hypothyroidism
Hyperthyroidism

Catecholamines
Testosterone
Primary sex characteristics
Secondary sex characteristics
Estrogen
Progesterone
Genetics
Behavior genetics
Extraversion
Neuroticism
Genes
Polygenetic
Chromosomes
Genotype
Phenotype
Genetic predisposition
Diathesis-stress model
Proband
Monozygotic (MZ) twins
Dizygotic (DZ) twins
Concordance

MATCHING

Match the following names, terms, and concepts with the definitions listed below. The answers are found at the end of the chapter.

a. self-efficacy expectations
b. psychosexual stages of development
c. self theory
d. magnification
e. ego
f. selective abstraction
g. observational learning
h. conditioned response
i. person variables
j. spontaneous recovery
k. limbic system
l. id
m. Aaron Beck

n. overgeneralization
o. Carl Jung
p. humanism
q. extinction
r. unconditional positive regard
s. superego
t. hierarchy of needs
u. Abraham Maslow
v. psychic structures
w. autonomic nervous system
x. personal constructs
y. Albert Ellis
z. unconditioned response

1) _____ psychic structure that follows the pleasures principle

2) _____ includes the id, ego, and superego

3) _____ neo-freudian who thought that our unconscious experience included archetypes

4) _____ psychic structure that follows the reality principle

5) _____ includes the oral, anal, phallic, latency, and genital stages

6) _____ psychic structure governed by the moral principle

7) _____ the recurrence of an extinguished CR, which results from the passage of time

8) _____ a response elicited by a stimulus without prior learning

9) _____ a response elicited by a CS as a result of a CS-US pairing

10) _____ an individual's beliefs about the likelihood of personal success at a task

11) _____ factors within an individual that must be considered in explaining behavior

12) _____ elimination of a CR by presentation of a CS alone

13) _____ acquisition of new behaviors by watching the performance of others

14) _____ developed cognitive therapy to help clients identify and correct cognitive errors

15) _____ developed rational emotive therapy

16) _____ the process of blowing unfortunate events out of proportion

17) _____ drawing broad conclusions from a few isolated events

18) _____ psychological dimensions by which we categorize ourselves, others, and our experiences

19) _____ focusing on personal flaws while ignoring competencies

20) _____ accepting the values of others regardless of the worth of their behavior at a particular time

21) _____ argued that people have growth-oriented needs for self-actualization

22) _____ focuses on the self as the executive of personality

23) _____ emerged as a third force in American psychology, in part a reaction to the prevailing psychodynamic and behavioral models

24) _____ a theory that ranges from basic biological needs to self-actualization needs

25) _____ this is divided into the sympathetic and parasympathetic branches

26) _____ a group of structures involved in memory, hunger, sex, and aggression

TRUE-FALSE

The following true-false statements are reprinted here from your text. Can you remember the answers? They can be found at the end of this chapter.

1. _____ According to psychodynamic theory, the mind is analogous to an immense iceberg; only the tip of it emerges into conscious awareness.
2. _____ Freud believed an ancient Greek legend about a king who slew his father and married his mother contained insights into the nature of human development.
3. _____ Researchers conditioned a young boy to fear rats by clanging steel bars behind his head while he played with a rat.
4. _____ Punishment does not work.
5. _____ People are more motivated to tackle arduous tasks if they believe they will succeed at them.
6. _____ People can make themselves miserable by the ways in which they interpret events.
7. _____ The risk of depression among Hispanic Americans is related to their level of acculturation to the mainstream U.S. culture.
8. _____ Abnormal behavior is connected with chemical imbalances in the brain.
9. _____ Anxiety can give you indigestion.
10. _____ Abnormal behavior patterns run in families.

MULTIPLE CHOICE

The multiple choice questions listed below will test your understanding of the material presented in the chapter. Read through each question and circle the letter representing the best answer. The answers are found at the end of the chapter.

1) Freud's structures of personality include:

    a. pleasure, reality, and moral
    b. id, ego, and superego
    c. unconscious, conscious, and preconscious
    d. oral, anal, phallic, latent, and genital

2) Freud is to Jung as:

    a. unconscious conflict is to archetype
    b. ego is to inferiority complex
    c. analytical psychology is to psychoanalytic theory
    c. psychoanalytic theory is to individual psychology

3) Which of the following ideas does not represent a major contribution of psychodynamic theory?

    a. defense mechanisms can distort our perceptions
    b. behavior can be motivated by hidden drives and impulses
    c. childhood experiences play a critical role in shaping abnormal behavior
    d. people have strong needs to reach their ego ideals

4) A student forgets that a difficult term paper is due. Which defense mechanism is at work?

    a. repression
    b. regression
    c. projection
    d. rationalization

5) Refusal to accept the true nature of a threat is the defense of:

    a. reaction formation
    b. denial
    c. sublimation
    d. displacement

6) Excessive self control and perfectionism may begin at which psychosexual stage?

    a. anal
    b. oral
    c. genital
    d. phallic

7) The learning perspective argues that abnormal behavior results from which of the following?

    a. double messages
    b. acting on irrational beliefs
    c. inappropriate or inadequate reinforcements
    d. unconscious conflict among learning experiences

8) In contrast to behaviorism, social learning theory emphasizes the importance of:

    a. conditioned stimuli as sources of fear
    b. confronting irrational beliefs
    c. goal setting and self-rewards
    d. consistent application of punishment

9) The major contributions of the learning perspective include which of the following?

    a. incorporating both environmental and unconscious variables into the search for causal relations in abnormal behavior
    b. emphasis on observable behavior and environmental stimuli
    c. emphasis on the critical learning experiences, which occur during the oral and anal stages of development
    d. a methodology for the experimental study of the collective unconscious

10) In the famous Pavlov study, which of the following was the conditioned stimulus (CS)?

    a. food
    b. salivation
    c. bell
    d. barking

11) In social learning theory, rewards and punishments represent which of the following?

    a. person variables
    b. encoding strategies
    c. expectations
    d. situation variables

12) All of the following contributed to the field of behaviorism EXCEPT:

    a. Aaron Beck
    b. John B. Watson
    c. B.F. Skinner
    d. Ivan Pavlov

13) All of the following are associated with cognitive theory EXCEPT:

    a. rational emotive therapy
    b. cognitive distortions
    c. individual psychology
    d. A-B-C approach

14) Many cognitive psychologists are influenced by concepts of:

    a. the unconscious
    b. computer science
    c. psychosexual development
    d. physics

15) Cognitive distortions refers to:

    a. errors in thinking
    b. aggression or hostility
    c. faulty processing
    d. impaired intellectual functioning

16) All of the following are psychodynamic theorists EXCEPT:

    a. Alfred Adler
    b. Karen Horney
    c. Harry Stack Sullivan
    d. Carl Rogers

17) In Erik Erikson's stages of development, the adolescent stage is characterized by the life crisis of:

    a. trust vs. mistrust
    b. identity vs. role diffusion
    c. autonomy vs. shame and doubt
    d. intimacy vs. isolation

18) Neurotic anxiety refers to:

    a. excessive feelings of guilt
    b. fear of external dangers or threats
    c. fear of one's own forbidden impulses
    d. the expression of primitive impulses

19) Who stressed the idea of personal constructs?

    a. Kelly
    b. Ellis
    c. Mahler
    d. Beck

20) The notion that adjustment is fostered by identification with both traditional and host countries is termed:

    a. bicultural theory
    b. melting pot theory
    c. logo theory
    d. social role theory

21) Operant conditioning occurs when an organism engages in a response and that response is:

    a. punished
    b. reinforced
    c. learned
    d. extinguished

22) A criticism of behaviorism is that:
    a. it lacks empirical validation
    b. it pays too much attention to genetic variation in explaining individual differences in behavior
    c. the emphasis placed on environmental or situational variables cannot be systematically varied or measured
    d. human behavior cannot be reduced to observable responses

23) The structure of a neuron which propagates messages over long distances is called a(n):

    a. synapse
    b. dendrite
    c. axon
    d. soma

24) Which of the following brain structures is associated with its function?

    a. the medulla is associated with balance and coordination
    b. the sympathetic nervous system is associated with eating
    c. the hypothalamus is associated with arousal and sleep
    d. the thalamus is associated with sensory relay

25) Dizziness, lack of energy, and trembling are symptoms of:

    a. hypoglycemia
    b. hyperglycemia
    c. hyperthyroidism
    d. anabolic steroid use

26) The diathesis-stress model of genetic-environment interaction suggests that:

    a. genotypic vulnerability combined with environmental stress yields abnormal behavior
    b. phenotypic vulnerability plus inappropriate learning yields abnormal behavior
    c. intrauterine, prenatal stress alters genotype to produce vulnerability
    d. genotypic vulnerability produces stress which yields abnormal behavior

27) Which of the following is NOT a major limitation to twin studies?

    a. the lack of access to adoption records
    b. the difficulty in finding MZ twins living in comparable socioeconomic classes to DZ twins
    c. MZ twins receiving greater encouragement to act alike
    d. finding MZ twins who were separated at birth

28) The nervous system is made up of nerve cells called:

    a. dendrites
    b. terminal buttons
    c. neurons
    d. knobs

29) All of the following are neurotransmitters EXCEPT:

    a. norepinephrine
    b. dopamine
    c. acetylcholine
    d. desipramine

30) The autonomic nervous system regulates all of the following activities EXCEPT:

    a. breathing
    b. walking
    c. heart rate
    d. digestion

QUESTIONS FOR CRITICAL THINKING

1. Contrast the function of the Id, Ego, and Superego.
2. Discuss how defense mechanisms can be both normal and abnormal.
3. Compare and contrast the psychosexual development of boys and girls according to Freud.
4. Discuss the strengths and weaknesses of the psychodynamic perspective.
5. How might fears become classically conditioned? How might you work with someone to get over a fear?
6. Compare and contrast operant conditioning and classical conditioning.
7. Evaluate the strengths and weaknesses of the learning perspective.
8. Discuss how cognitive theorists compare you and I to computers.
9. Discuss the strengths and weaknesses of the cognitive perspective.
10. Discuss the effect that Nazi horrors had on Viktor Frankl.
11. Discuss the complaints that humanists have about psychodynamic and behavioral theories. Do you agree or disagree and why?
12. Discuss the strengths and weaknesses of humanistic-existential theories.
13. Discuss the general findings on acculturation and psychological disorders. What might explain the inconsistencies in these findings?
14. Discuss the role neurotransmitters might play in abnormal behavior.
15. Compare and contrast kinship and twin studies.
16. Discuss the strengths and weaknesses of the biological perspective.
17. If you were planning to see a psychotherapist for depression, which perspective would you feel the most comfortable with? What about for a phobia?

ANSWERS FOR MATCHING

1.	l	10.	a	19.	f
2.	v	11.	i	20.	r
3.	o	12.	q	21.	u
4.	e	13.	g	22.	c
5.	b	14.	m	23.	p
6.	s	15.	y	24.	t
7.	j	16.	d	25.	w
8.	z	17.	n	26.	k
9.	h	18.	x		

TRUE-FALSE ANSWERS

1.	T	6.	T
2.	T	7.	T
3.	T	8.	T
4.	F	9.	T
5.	T	10.	T

MULTIPLE CHOICE ANSWERS

1.	b	11.	d	21.	b
2.	a	12.	a	22.	d
3.	d	13.	c	23.	c
4.	a	14.	b	24.	d
5.	b	15.	a	25.	a
6.	a	16.	d	26.	a
7.	c	17.	b	27.	b
8.	c	18.	c	28.	c
9.	b	19.	a	29.	d
10.	c	20.	a	30.	b

CHAPTER THREE

CLASSIFICATION AND ASSESSMENT OF ABNORMAL BEHAVIOR

OVERVIEW

While the previous chapters have provided a general perspective on abnormal behavior and research methods, this chapter moves closer to abnormal behavior, looking not so much at the larger picture, but at the methods we use to assess and classify abnormal behavior. The DSM classification system is presented first. It represents a framework used by the medical and psychological communities. Major portions of this textbook are organized around DSM groupings of disorders.

After reviewing issues of reliability and validity as they apply to psychological tests, the chapter focuses on approaches to clinical interviewing and three major types of tests: intelligence tests, personality tests, and neuropsychological assessment instruments. The final sections of the chapter present other assessment methods in the behavioral and cognitive areas as well as some emerging technology in direct physiological measurement and medical imaging. You should view all of these assessment methods as a relatively comprehensive tool kit for assessing abnormal behavior. Generally, information from several of these methods is gathered and assembled before an individual is classified in the DSM system.

CHAPTER OUTLINE

Classification of Abnormal Behavior
The DSM and Models of Abnormal Behavior
     Features of the DSM
         The DSM-IV
     Evaluation of the DSM System
     Advantages and Disadvantages of the DSM System
     Sociocultural Factors in the Classification of Abnormal Behavior
Characteristics of Methods of Assessment
     Reliability
         Internal Consistency
         Temporal Stability
         Interrater Reliability
     Validity
         Content Validity
         Criterion Validity
         Construct Validity
     Sociocultural and Ethnic Factors in the Assessment of Abnormal Behavior
The Clinical Interview
     Mental Status Examination

LEARNING OBJECTIVES

The following learning objectives can also be found at the beginning of the chapter. When you have completed your study of the chapter, you should be able to:

1. Discuss historical origins of modern diagnostic systems.
2. Define the concept of "mental disorders" in the DSM system and show how the diagnostic system adheres to the medical model.
3. Describe the features of the DSM system.
4. Explain the multiaxial feature of the DSM.
5. Describe the strengths and weaknesses of the DSM system.

6. Discuss the sociocultural and ethnic factors in the classification of abnormal behavior.
7. Explain three approaches to demonstrating the reliability of methods of assessment.
8. Explain three approaches to demonstrating the validity of methods of assessment.
9. Discuss sociocultural and ethnic factors in the assessment of abnormal behavior.
10. Describe what is meant by a structured interview.
11. Describe the elements of the mental status examination.
12. Describe the use of standardized interview techniques.
13. Discuss the nature and value of psychological tests.
14. Discuss the history and features of the Stanford-Binet Intelligence Scale.
15. Discuss the features of the Wechsler Scales.
16. Distinguish between self-report and projective personality assessment techniques.
17. Discuss the history, features, reliability, and validity of personality tests, focusing on the MMPI and the Rorschach.
18. Explain how various response sets can distort test results.
19. Describe the use of psychological tests in the assessment of neuropsychological functioning.
20. Discuss the advantages and limitations of behavioral assessments.
21. Describe the following techniques: the behavioral interview, self-monitoring, use of contrived measures, direct observation, and behavioral rating scales.
22. Discuss the use of thought diaries and questionnaires that assess automatic thoughts and dysfunctional attitudes.
23. Explain the relationships between emotional states and physiological measurement.
24. Describe contemporary brain-imaging techniques.

KEY TERMS AND CONCEPTS

The following is a list of terms, concepts, and names that are discussed in the chapter. They are important for you to know. Review these terms, comparing your answers with the material presented in the text.

Hippocrates
Emil Kraeplin
Diagnostic and Statistical Manual (DSM)
International Classification of Diseases (ICD)
Neurosis
Mental disorder

Diagnostic criteria
Essential features
Associated features
Multiaxial
Syndromes
Principal diagnosis
Reliability
Validity
Predictive validity
Diagnosis
Sanism
Culture-bound syndromes
Internal consistency
Coefficient alpha
Temporal stability
Test-retest reliability
Interrater reliability
Content validity
Criterion validity
Concurrent validity
Sensitivity
Specificity
False negative
False positive
Predictive validity
Construct validity
Phrenologists
Intake interview
Presenting problem
Structured interview
Rapport
Mental status examination
Orientation
Sensorium
Affect
Mood
Standardized interview
Closed-ended questions
Open-ended questions
Intelligence
Alfred Binet
Theodore Simon
Mental age
Louis Terman
Intelligence quotient

Deviation IQ
David Wechsler
Self-report
Projective test
Objective test
Forced-choice format
Starke Hathaway
Charles McKinley
Contrasted groups approach
Validity scales
Standard scores
Content scales
Projective tests
Hermann Rorschach
Inquiry
Reality testing
Henry Murray
Apperception
Neuropsychologist
False negative
Psychometric approach
Behavioral assessment
Analogues
Functional analysis
Behavioral interview
Self-monitoring
Baseline
Reactivity
Observer drift
Behavioral rating scale
Electrodermal response
Galvanic skin response
Electroencephalograph
Electromyograph
Ambulatory blood pressure
Computerized axial tomography
Positron emission tomography
Magnetic resonance imaging

MATCHING

Match the following names, terms, and concepts with the definitions listed below. The answers are found at the end of the chapter.

a. developmental disorders
b. insight
c. concurrent validity
d. analogue measures
e. validity
f. deviation IQ
g. general medical conditions
h. functional analysis
i. criterion validity
j. structured interview
k. rapport
l. coefficient alpha
m. electroencephalograph

n. interrater reliability
o. presenting problem
p. Hermann Rorschach
q. thought process
r. validity scales
s. temporal stability
t. behavioral rating scale
u. Louis Terman
v. sensorium
w. reactivity
x. diagnostic criteria
y. reliability
z. intake interview

1) _____ part of Axis II, includes mental retardation

2) _____ consistency of measurement

3) _____ behavioral change resulting from being observed

4) _____ extent to which client understands and recognizes his or her problem

5) _____ checklist of behaviors that provides information about frequency and intensity

6) _____ relationship of assessment responses to an external standard

7) _____ adapted the Binet-Simon for use with American children

8) _____ Axis III of DSM, conditions that may affect functioning or response to treatment

9) _____ finding relationship of behavior to its antecedents and consequences

10) _____ complaint that leads client to seek therapy

11) _____ a measure of internal consistency

12) _____ observations made in role-playing situations

13) _____ retesting yields similar results

14) _____ client's form and content of thought

15) _____ MMPI scales that detect clients trying to "fake good" or "fake bad"

16) _____ feelings of trust between therapist and client

17) _____ noninvasive measurement of electrical activity of brain

18) _____ developed projective test using inkblots as stimuli

19) _____ measurements correspond to what they are intended to assess

20) _____ level of agreement between two or more judges

21) _____ judgments about client's focusing of attention and capacity for concentration

22) _____ an IQ measure based on deviation from norms of an age group

23) _____ a standard series of questions are asked to obtain clinically useful information

24) _____ diagnostic anchors that define particular patterns of abnormal behavior

25) _____ initial interview to learn about client's presenting problem and history

26) _____ extent to which an assessment device predicts scores on a second measuring device

TRUE-FALSE

The following true-false statements are reprinted here from your text. Can you remember the answers? They can be found at the end of the chapter.

1. _____ A psychological test can be highly reliable yet also invalid.
2. _____ Researchers find that people report more personal problems when interviewed by computers than by humans.
3. _____ An IQ score of 130 puts you in the genius category.
4. _____ A widely used personality test is composed of items that were answered in the same direction by people with psychological disorders and normal groups.
5. _____ Some clinicians form diagnostic impressions on the basis of how clients interpret inkblots.

6. _____ Clients can be fitted with equipment that allows clinicians to measure their physiological responses as they go about their daily lives.

7. _____ Despite advances in medicine, surgery remains the only available means of probing the workings of the brain.

MULTIPLE CHOICE

The multiple choice questions listed below will test your understanding of the material presented in the chapter. Read through each question and circle the letter representing the best answer. The answers are found at the end of the chapter.

1) The DSM classification system is an outgrowth of the work of:

    a. Henry Murray
    b. Emil Kraeplin
    c. Hippocrates
    d. Sigmund Freud

2) A client is recording the situation surrounding emotional states, and the category of disordered thinking that accompanied the emotional state. This client is using:

    a. a personality inventory
    b. contrived measures
    c. a thought diary
    d. direct observation

3) Questions in the MMPI:

    a. are open ended
    b. were selected because they discriminated between normal and clinical diagnostic populations
    c. were selected to detect individuals trying to "fake good"
    d. were chosen because they have a single correct answer

4) The major value of the standardized interview is in:

    a. its ability to produce high reliability without special training of interviewers
    b. minimizing interview time
    c. validity of diagnostic classification
    d. reliability of diagnostic classification

5) Which of the following is NOT an advantage of classification?

    a. it helps researchers identify populations with similar patterns of abnormal behavior
    b. it helps clinicians predict behavior
    c. being labelled makes clients feel better
    d. it fosters communication between researchers

6) Which brain-imaging technique requires a person to be placed In a tunnel that generates a strong magnetic field?

    a. MRI
    b. CAT scan
    c. PET scan
    d. BEAM

7) Lang suggested that fear or anxiety consists of three different response systems:

    a. cognitive, emotional, and physiological
    b. conscious, unconscious, and preconscious
    c. behavioral, physiological, and verbal
    d. behavioral, cognitive, and subconscious

8) Performance on which test of the Halstead-Reitan Neuropsychological Battery is believed to reflect functioning in the frontal lobe of the brain?

    a. category
    b. rhythm
    c. motor skills
    d. tactile performance

9) That people with bipolar disorder as diagnosed by DSM respond well to lithium supports the DSM's:

    a. temporal stability
    b. diagnostic "purity"
    c. coverage
    d. predictive validity

10) The Automatic Thoughts Questionnaire is an example of:

    a. a cognitive assessment measure
    b. a behavioral assessment measure
    c. a personality assessment measure
    d. a standardized interview

11) Specific diagnostic criteria in DSM-IV:

    a. include essential features and associated features
    b. group behaviors according to their underlying causes
    c. are largely grouped according to psychodynamic theory
    d. are explanatory rather than descriptive

12) Patterns of abnormal behavior that impair functioning and are stressful to the individual are coded on which DSM axis?

    a. I
    b. II
    c. III
    d. IV

13) Criterion validity has two general types:

    a. content and concurrent
    b. construct and content
    c. construct and predictive
    d. concurrent and predictive

14) A projective test that requires people to respond to an ambiguous scene by constructing a story is:

    a. MMPI
    b. MCMI
    c. TAT
    d. Rorschach

15) On the Rorschach, what is an index of reality testing?

    a. form
    b. color
    c. movement
    d. location

16) Problems with the use of direct observation include all but which of the following?

    a. lack of consensus in defining problems in behavioral terms
    b. measuring only private experiences
    c. reactivity
    d. observer drift

17) Which of the following is a major advantage of DSM?

     a. it eliminates multiple diagnosis
     b. high validity
     c. low reliability
     d. it develops a comprehensive view as a result of its multiaxial system

18) A clinician who asks a series of questions about problem behaviors, their histories, and their relationship to situational events is using which method of assessment?

     a. the mental status examination
     b. self-monitoring
     c. a behavioral checklist
     d. the behavioral interview

19) Research on sociocultural and ethnic factors in assessment of personality functioning suggests that:

     a. if they are translated correctly, assessment techniques are reliable and valid
     b. adequate norms for diagnostic instruments are available for all cultural and ethnic groups
     c. cultural differences must be taken into account when making diagnostic judgements
     d. semantic factors in diagnostic instruments do not account for any differences in rates of depression across countries

20) A mental disorder (in DSM) requires:

     a. statistically uncommon behavior
     b. an expected response to a stressful event
     c. emotional distress or impaired functioning
     d. demonstration of a biological cause

21) A disadvantage of self-rating scales is that:

     a. they are costly to administer
     b. many clients find them difficult to complete because of their complexity
     c. good interrater reliability is difficult to achieve
     d. because they rely on clients as the source of data, the test responses may be biased in some way

22) Questions such as "Would you please tell me your name?" and "Do you know what the date is today?" help assess:

    a. mood
    b. orientation
    c. insight
    d. judgement

23) An advantage of the Wechsler intelligence scales is:

    a. an examiner is not necessary because all of the tests are self-report
    b. questions are age-graded
    c. a persons "mental age" can be determined
    d. relative strengths and weaknesses of a person are assessed, not just an overall score

24) Which assessment method has the advantage of not relying on clients' self-reports but which may be distorted by attempts by the client to make a positive impression?

    a. self-monitoring using a wrist counter
    b. direct observation
    c. the behavioral rating scale
    d. measurement of the electrodermal response

25) The degree to which a test correctly identifies people who have a particular disorder is:

    a. sensitivity
    b. face validity
    c. specificity
    d. false positive

26) An advantage of the DSM-IV is:

    a. it does not rely on the medical model
    b. it only includes "culture-free" disorders
    c. it is more strongly based on empirical evidence than earlier versions
    d. it represents a completely different approach to classifying abnormal behavior than earlier versions

27) Which of the following would be coded on Axis IV of the DSM-IV?

    a. a personality disorder
    b. diabetes
    c. problems related to the social environment
    d. the clinician's judgment of the client's overall functioning

28) An example of a culture-bound syndrome is:

    a. mental retardation
    b. depression
    c. anorexia nervosa
    d. schizophrenia

29) An electromyograph measures:

    a. brain waves
    b. muscle tension
    c. sweating
    d. brain density

30) The psychometric approach holds that:

    a. projective tests are currently the most reliable assessment devices in order to predict people's behavior
    b. psychological tests reveal signs of reasonably stable traits or dispositions that largely determine people's behavior
    c. only standardized instruments should be used to determine personality functioning
    d. samples of behavior are the most accurate method of determining people's behavior

QUESTIONS FOR CRITICAL THINKING

1. How does the DSM adhere to the medical model?
2. How do sociocultural and ethnic factors affect classification of abnormal behavior?
3. Discuss why assessing the validity of diagnostic categories is so complex.
4. What are culture-bound disorders?
5. When is test-retest reliability especially important?
6. How do concurrent and predictive validity differ?
7. How might an interviewer's theoretical framework influence the clinical interview?
8. How effective are computers at interviewing?

9. Discuss the components of a mental status interview.
10. Compare the use of a structured interview such as the SCID to a clinical interview. What are the advantages and disadvantages of each?
11. Why was the MMPI-2 developed?
12. What are the strengths and weaknesses of the Rorschach and the TAT?
13. Compare and contrast the Halstead-Reitan and the Luria-Nebraska test batteries.
14. Discuss the advantages and limitations of behavioral assessment.
15. Discuss the use of thought diaries and questionnaires that assess automatic thoughts and dysfunctional attitudes.
16. Explain the relationships between emotional states and physiological measurement.
17. Describe contemporary brain-imaging techniques.

ANSWERS FOR MATCHING

1.	a	10.	o	19.	e
2.	y	11.	l	20.	n
3.	w	12.	d	21.	v
4.	b	13.	s	22.	f
5.	t	14.	q	23.	j
6.	i	15.	r	24.	x
7.	u	16.	k	25.	z
8.	g	17.	m	26.	c
9.	h	18.	p		

TRUE-FALSE ANSWERS

1.	T	5.	T
2.	T	6.	T
3.	F	7.	F
4.	F		

MULTIPLE CHOICE ANSWERS

1.	b	11.	a	21.	d
2.	c	12.	a	22.	b
3.	b	13.	d	23.	d
4.	d	14.	c	24.	b
5.	c	15.	a	25.	a
6.	a	16.	b	26.	c
7.	c	17.	d	27.	c
8.	a	18.	d	28.	c
9.	d	19.	c	29.	b
10.	a	20.	c	30.	b

CHAPTER FOUR

METHODS OF THERAPY AND TREATMENT

OVERVIEW

The text chapter opens by developing a definition of what psychotherapy is. The chapter continues by describing the following four major types of psychologically-based psychotherapy is separate sections: Psychodynamic Therapies, Humanistic-Existential Therapies, Cognitive Therapies, and Behavior Therapy. We call these therapies "psychological" because they look for causes and treatment for abnormal behavior in the feelings, thoughts, and behavior of the individual instead of attempting to understand abnormal behavior through biological explanations.

Traditionally, psychotherapy has been focused on the individual, however, there are alternative methods for treatment. Therefore, after examining the four major psychological psychotherapies, your chapter examines Group Therapy as well as Family and Marital Therapy. The analysis of psychological psychotherapies ends with the consideration of an extremely controversial topic, the effectiveness of psychotherapy.

Your text also explores Multicultural Issues in Psychotherapy and examines issues related specifically to African Americans, Asian Americans, Hispanic Americans, and Native Americans. In addition, your chapter examines Biological Therapies, which include chemotherapy, electroconvulsive therapy (ECT), and psychosurgery. This final section of the chapter examines issues related to deinstitutionalization and state mental hospitals as well as community-based care.

CHAPTER OUTLINE

Psychotherapy
 Major Types of Mental Health Professionals
  Clinical Psychologists
  Psychiatrists
  Psychiatric Social Workers
 Traditional Psychoanalysis
  Free Association
  Dream Analysis
  Transference
 Modern Psychodynamic Approaches
Humanistic-Existential Therapies
 Person-Centered Therapy
 Existential Therapies
Cognitive Therapies
 Rational-Emotive Therapy
 Beck's Cognitive Therapy

LEARNING OBJECTIVES

The following learning objectives can also be found at the beginning of the chapter. When you have completed your study of the chapter, you should be able to:

1. Define psychotherapy.
2. Describe the goals and methods of traditional psychoanalysis.
3. Compare and contrast traditional psychoanalysis with modern psychodynamic approaches.
4. Describe the philosophies and goals of humanistic-existential therapies.
5. Describe the methods of person-centered therapy and existential therapies.
6. Describe the philosophies and goals of cognitive therapies.
7. Compare and contrast the methods of rational-emotive therapy with Beck's cognitive therapy.
8. Describe the philosophy and goals of behavior therapy.
9. Describe systematic desensitization, gradual exposure, aversive conditioning, operant conditioning, social skills training, and methods for fostering self-control.
10. Discuss the development of eclectic approaches in psychotherapy.
11. Describe the advantages of group therapy.
12. Describe psychodrama and encounter groups.
13. Describe marital and family therapy approaches.
14. Discuss the problems in attempting to evaluate the effectiveness of psychotherapy in direct comparisons between different therapies.
15. Explain the technique of meta-analysis.
16. Summarize the findings of research into the effectiveness of psychotherapy in general and specific therapeutic approaches in particular.
17. Discuss issues relating to the use of traditional Western psychotherapy approaches with diverse cultural and racial groups.
18. Discuss treatment techniques that are aimed at ethnic minority groups.
19. Describe the uses and abuses of drug therapy.
20. Describe electroconvulsive therapy and psychosurgery and explain why these techniques are controversial.
21. Discuss ethnic factors in the utilization of mental-health services.
22. Describe the contemporary roles of the community mental-health center and the mental hospital.
23. Discuss the outcomes of deinstitutionalization and the problems of the psychiatric homeless population.

KEY TERMS AND CONCEPTS

The following is a list of terms, concepts, and names that are discussed in the chapter. They are important for you to know. Review these terms, comparing your answers with the material presented in the text.

Psychotherapy
Placebo effects
Expectancy effects
Nonspecific factors
Clinical psychologists
Psychiatrists
Psychiatric social workers
Psychoanalysis
Interpretation
Free association
Resistance
Insight
Manifest content
Latent content
Displacing
Transference relationship
Transference neurosis
Countertransference
Ego analysts
Melanie Klein
Margaret Mahler
Object-relations
Carl Rogers
Person-centered therapy
Unconditional positive regard
Empathic understanding
Genuineness
Congruence
Ludwig Binswanger
Medard Boss
Viktor Frankl
Rollo May
Albert Ellis
Aaron Beck
Cognitive therapy
Cognitive distortions
Behavior therapy
Behavior modification
Systematic desensitization

Gradual exposure
Modeling
Albert Bandura
Aversive conditioning
Operant conditioning
Token economy
Social skills training
Assertiveness training
Functional analysis
Eclecticism
Technical eclectics
Integrative eclectics
Group therapy
Family therapy
Virginia Satir
Structural family therapy
Marital therapy
Spontaneous remission
Meta-analysis
Therapeutic alliance
Working alliance
Cultural responsiveness hypothesis
Cuento therapy
Feminist therapy
Biological psychiatry
Psychopharmacology
Antianxiety drugs
Rebound anxiety
Antipsychotic drugs/major tranquilizers/neuroleptics
Antidepressants
Tricyclics
Monoamine oxidase (MAO) inhibitors
Selective serotonin-reuptake inhibitors (SSRIs)
Electroconvulsive therapy (ECT)
Prefrontal lobotomy
Antonio Egas Moniz
Deinstitutionalization
Community mental-health centers (CMHCs)

MATCHING

Match the following names, terms, and concepts with the definitions listed below. The answers are found at the end of the chapter.

a. Albert Ellis
b. deinstitutionalization
c. self-control techniques
d. latent content
e. antidepressants
f. chemotherapy
g. existential therapy
h. Virginia Satir
i. cognitive therapy
j. clinical psychologist
k. psychodrama
l. token economy
m. operant conditioning

n. meta analysis
o. interpretation
p. modeling
q. encounter groups
r. major tranquilizers
s. systematic desensitization
t. manifest content
u. cuento therapy
v. antianxiety drugs
w. Carl Rogers
x. community mental-health centers
y. resistance
z. psychiatrist

1) _____ Ph.D. trained in the assessment, diagnosis, and treatment of mental disorders

2) _____ the unconscious material symbolized by dream content

3) _____ the content of a dream that a dreamer experiences

4) _____ M.D. or D.O. with a residency in diagnosis and treatment of mental disorders

5) _____ the founder of client-centered therapy

6) _____ in psychoanalytic theory, a psychoanalyst will offer this as a way to draw the client's attention to connections between disclosures and unconscious conflicts

7) _____ a therapeutic orientation that stresses the importance of coming to terms with the fundamental question of existence

8) _____ the founder of rational-emotive therapy

9) _____ a therapeutic orientation that focuses on changing maladaptive thoughts into more accurate ones

10) _____ using observational learning to treat phobias

11) _____ using reinforcement principles to learn adaptive behaviors

12) _____ examples of this include assertiveness training, self-monitoring, modeling, and behavior rehearsal

13) _____ combines muscle relaxation with imagination of phobic stimuli

14) _____ a system of applying operant conditioning principles to institutions

15) _____ a type of group therapy THAT seeks to foster self-awareness

16) _____ conflict re-enactment in a group therapy context

17) _____ theorist who conceptualized the family in terms of a pattern or system of communications and interactions that needs to be studied and changed to enhance family and individual functioning

18) _____ a statistical technique for averaging the results of large numbers of studies

19) _____ according to psychoanalytic theory, this is an unwillingness or inability to recall or discuss disturbing or threatening material

20) _____ prescribing medication as treatment for abnormal behavior

21) _____ shifting mental health care from hospitals to the community

22) _____ medication used to treat hallucinations, delusions, and confusion states

23) _____ an example of this might be a series of videotaped vignettes presented to clients in order to convey culturally-laden messages intended to relate a specific message

24) _____ drugs that depress the level of activity in certain parts of the central nervous system

25) _____ include tricyclics, monoamine oxidase (MAO) inhibitors, and selective serotonin-reuptake inhibitors (SSRIs)

26) _____ perform many functions in the effort to reduce the need for hospitalization or re-hospitalization

TRUE-FALSE

The following true-false statements are reprinted here from your text. Can you remember the answers? They can be found at the end of this chapter.

1. _____ In some states, anyone can set up shop as a psychotherapist.
2. _____ Some therapists ask clients to lie down on a couch and express whatever thoughts come to mind.
3. _____ Some therapists believe negative emotions like anxiety and depression are not directly caused by troubling events that people experience, but rather by the ways in which they interpret events.
4. _____ Group therapy is less expensive than individual therapy, but individual therapy is preferable for clients who can afford it.
5. _____ Despite the claims made by therapists, little scientific evidence supports the effectiveness of psychotherapy.
6. _____ A psychotic Haitian man responded positively to a form of therapy that included the lifting of a curse by a *voodoo* priest.
7. _____ Electroconvulsive therapy is helpful in many cases of depression that do not respond to other forms of therapy.
8. _____ Although some ex-hospitalized psychiatric patients have fallen through the cracks of the mental-health system, the vast majority are receiving the support they need to function effectively in the community.

MULTIPLE CHOICE

The multiple choice questions listed below will test your understanding of the material presented in the chapter. Read through each question and circle the letter representing the best answer. The answers are found at the end of the chapter.

1) Which of the following is NOT one of the defining characteristics of psychotherapy?

    a. psychotherapy involves the use of psychological principles, research, and theory
    b. psychotherapy can relieve abnormal behavior, develop problem solving skills, and promote personal growth
    c. psychotherapy changes behavior, thoughts, and feelings
    d. psychotherapy involves a core fundamental system of interaction utilized by all therapeutic orientations

2) A therapist is having trouble at home with his or her spouse. Soon, the therapist begins arguing more and more with clients. This could be an example of:

   a. manifest content
   b. resistance
   c. countertransference
   c. transference

3) Modern psychodynamic approaches are _____ than traditional psychoanalysis.

   a. more ambiguous
   b. less effective
   c. less respected
   d. more ego focused

4) Which of the following is NOT an appropriate question to ask while choosing a psychologist to work with?

   a. "What are your areas of expertise?"
   b. "Could you prescribe medication for my problem?"
   c. "What experience do you have helping people with my type of problem?"
   d. "What kinds of treatments do you use?"

5) Which of the following is the process of uttering uncensored thoughts as they come to mind?

   a. free association
   b. interpretation
   c. chunking
   d. insight

6) Humanistic-existential approaches to therapy differ from psychoanalytic approaches by:

   a. emphasizing the past
   b. trying to achieve insight
   c. emphasizing conscious conflicts
   d. trying to overcome congruence

7) If the therapist asks a client to confront opposing elements in his or her personality, the therapist is attempting to establish which of the following:

    a. congruence
    b. dialogue
    c. empathetic understanding
    d. genuineness

8) According to cognitive therapies, which of the following is true:

    a. abnormal feelings produce abnormal behavior
    b. unconscious thoughts produce abnormal behavior
    c. awareness of childhood conflict leads to adaptive adult behavior
    d. maladaptive, automatic thoughts produce abnormal behavior

9) . All of the following are examples of cognitive distortions EXCEPT:

    a. saying "she seems very upset with me" after a fight with a friend
    b. selectively perceiving only one's flaws
    c. saying "no one will ever ask me out again" after a break-up with a partner
    d. focusing on negative outcomes and ignoring the positive

10) Asking a client to act inconsistently with their beliefs to check their accuracy is called:

    a. behavior modification
    b. flooding
    c. reality testing
    d. congruence checking

11) Which of the following is most likely to be a treatment goal of a behavior therapist dealing with a depressed person?

    a. helping the client to develop a positive self image
    b. gain insight into troubling, sibling conflict
    c. uncover childhood trauma leading to the depression
    d. increase the frequency of getting out the house

12) During the 1940's and 1950's, most psychotherapists were:

    a. eclectic
    b. psychodynamic
    c. person-centered
    d. behavioral

13) Which of the following first gained widespread attention as a means of helping people overcome fears and phobias?

    a. cognitive therapy
    b. behavior therapy
    c. psychoanalysis
    d. humanistic therapy

14) Fear-reduction methods of treatment instill _____ behaviors, while aversive conditioning leads to the development of _____ behaviors.

    a. approach; avoidance
    b. avoidance; approach
    c. adaptive; maladaptive
    d. maladaptive; adaptive

15) Which of the following pioneered modeling techniques?

    a. Albert Ellis
    b. Carl Rogers
    c. Albert Bandura
    d. B.F. Skinner

16) Which of the following refers to a systematic study of an antecedent stimuli of a problem behavior and the reinforcers that maintain that behavior?

    a. operant conditioning
    b. functional analysis
    c. token economy
    d. classical conditioning

17) Which of the following statements is NOT true about group therapy?

    a. group therapy is more efficient because more people can be treated at one time
    b. groups are especially useful in treating problems involving social interactions
    c. therapist support in a group setting may be more powerful than peer support in increasing self-esteem
    d. group therapy provides the opportunity for learning to deal more effectively with other people

18) Encounter groups represent a group therapy technique developed by which type of therapy?

    a. Humanistic-Existential
    b. Cognitive
    c. Behavioral
    d. Psychodynamic

19) Which of the following is most likely a goal of a structural family therapist:

    a. working individually with the identified patient to provide coping strategies for dealing effectively with dysfunctional family patterns
    b. analyzing family roles played by individual members and helping families to restructure themselves in ways that are more supportive of the members
    c. working with the family to reframe negative events and interactions more positively
    d. analyzing childhood trauma of the identified patient and how that affects his or her interactions with family members

20) A humanistic-existential therapist would accept which of the following as an appropriate outcome measure?

    a. direct observation of the problem behavior
    b. changes in EEG and GSR measures
    c. reports from a work supervisor related to the client's behavior
    d. client's report of how they feel

21) Your textbook suggests that, in general, research evidence indicates that psychotherapy:

    a. is effective
    b. is not effective
    c. is effective for a limited number of individuals
    d. may be effective, but we cannot tell from present research evidence

22) Evidence regarding the psychological treatment of low-income groups and people of color indicate that:

    a. psychotherapy is helpful regardless of cultural sensitivity of the therapist
    b. psychotherapy is helpful when treatment is offered in a culturally sensitive context
    c. psychotherapy is helpful only when the therapist is of the same cultural background as the client
    d. psychotherapy is essentially unsuccessful with low-income groups and people of color

23) The cultural responsiveness hypothesis suggests that:

    a. clients will respond to therapy only if the therapist addresses issues related to culture and ethnicity
    b. clients will not respond to therapy if the therapist has no knowledge about their ethnic background
    c. clients will respond better to therapy when the therapist is similar to them in ethnic and language background
    d. ethnic and cultural issues related to the therapist is not a factor for clients who identify strongly with their own culture

24) All of the following may deter Asian Americans from recognizing problems and seeking help to deal with them EXCEPT:

    a. the therapist may be viewed as an authority type which may conflict with their preference to clarify their feelings and reach their own decisions
    b. mental-health problems carry a severe social stigma
    c. the emphasis in Western psychotherapy on the open expression of feelings may conflict with traditional Asian tendencies to refrain from public displays of emotion
    d. they may prefer structured, unambiguous approaches to solving problems rather than the open-ended, unstructured style of Western insight-oriented psychotherapies

25) Which of the following is NOT TRUE of feminist therapy?

    a. it emerged as a response to male dominance of mental-health professions and institutions
    b. it challenges the tendency of traditional psychotherapies to label as normal those attributes identified with the male-dominated mainstream culture
    c. it contends that traditional therapies label any behaviors that do not serve the interests of minorities groups as problematic
    d. it challenges the use of gender-role stereotypes to support cultural beliefs in male superiority and female inferiority

26) Phenothiazines like Thorazine are used to treat:

    a. anxiety disorders
    b. depression
    c. psychosis (hallucinations and delusions)
    d. sleeping disorders

27) ECT remains a controversial treatment for depression because:

    a. there is no clear evidence that it is more effective than antidepressant
       medication
    b. one of ECT's side effects is permanent memory loss
    c. it is not clear how or why it works
    d. all of the above statements are true

28) The nerve that joins the _____ and the _____ _ is severed in a
prefrontal lobotomy.

    a. prefrontal cortex; frontal cortex
    b. thalamus; prefrontal cortex
    c. hypothalamus; thalamus
    d. frontal cortex; caudal cortex

29) All of the following are antianxiety medications EXCEPT:

    a. prozac
    b. valium
    c. xanax
    d. librium

30) Which of the following is true of selective serotonin-reuptake inhibitors (SSRIs)?

    a. they increase the availability of serotonin and decrease the availability of
       norepinephrine in the brain
    b. they decrease the availability of serotonin in the brain
    c. they increase the availability of serotonin in the brain
    d. they decrease the availability of serotonin and increase the availability of
       norepinephrine in the brain

QUESTIONS FOR CRITICAL THINKING

1.   Discuss why anyone seeking help for psychological problems should ask about
       the therapist's training.
2.   Compare and contrast transference and countertransference.
3.   Discuss how modern psychodynamic approaches differ from traditional
       methods.
4.   Discuss non-directive therapy. What are the reasons behind a therapist using
       this approach to treatment?
5.   Compare and contrast behavioral, cognitive, humanistic-existential,
       psychodynamic, and biological approaches to treatment.

6. Discuss how the goals of self control technique differ from that of insight therapy.
7. Provide an example of how a therapist might use eclecticism to treat a client with depression.
8. Compare and contrast group therapy with individual therapy. What are the advantages and disadvantages   of each?
9. Discuss the cultural responsiveness hypothesis.
10. Discuss the methodological problems in comparing different therapeutic approaches.
11. Identify and discuss the empirically validated psychological treatments that have been demonstrated to be effective for treating bulimia, institutionalized populations, specific phobias, enuresis, and generalized anxiety disorder.
12. Discuss the tenets of feminist therapy.
13. Discuss the therapy approaches that have been useful with non-white ethnic populations.
14. Discuss why ECT is a controversial treatment for depression.
15. Discuss the issues related to the underutilization of mental-health services by ethnic groups.
16. Discuss the advantages and disadvantages of deinstitutionalization.

ANSWERS FOR MATCHING

1.	j	10.	p	19.	y
2.	d	11.	m	20.	f
3.	t	12.	c	21.	b
4.	z	13.	s	22.	r
5.	w	14.	l	23.	u
6.	o	15.	q	24.	v
7.	g	16.	k	25.	e
8.	a	17.	h	26.	x
9.	i	18.	n		

TRUE-FALSE ANSWERS

1.	T	5.	F
2.	T	6.	T
3.	T	7.	T
4.	F	8.	F

MULTIPLE CHOICE ANSWERS

1.	d	11.	d	21.	a
2.	c	12.	b	22.	b
3.	d	13.	b	23.	c
4.	b	14.	a	24.	a
5.	a	15.	c	25.	c
6.	c	16.	b	26.	c
7.	b	17.	c	27.	d
8.	d	18.	a	28.	b
9.	a	19.	b	29.	a
10.	c	20.	d	30.	c

CHAPTER FIVE

STRESS, PSYCHOLOGICAL FACTORS, AND HEALTH

OVERVIEW

This chapter describes how stress and psychological factors can combine to influence our health. The first section describes adjustment disorders and explains how stress can be related to illness. Next, the authors present a multifactorial view of the health-illness spectrum. Among these factors are biological and psychological variables. Additional elements include socioeconomic, sociocultural, and ethnic factors, as well as natural environmental and technology-produced factors. The final, and largest section of the chapter considers the relation of psychological factors to a wide variety of illnesses and conditions. Among these are headaches, cardiovascular disorders, digestive problems, asthma, and obesity. The chapter also discusses psychological elements in two very deadly disorders, cancer and AIDS. Finally, the chapter identifies physiological and psychological factors related to sleep disorders.

CHAPTER OUTLINE

Adjustment Disorders
    Stress and Illness
        The Immune System
        Stress and the Immune System
    Stress and Life Changes
        The General Adaptation Syndrome
A Multifactorial View of Health and Illness
    Biological Factors
    Psychological Factors
        Self-Efficacy Expectancies
        Psychological Hardiness
        Optimism
        Humor: Does "A Merry Heart Doeth Good Like a Medicine?"
    Socioeconomic, Sociocultural, and Ethnic Factors
        Social Support
        Mediators of Stress among African Americans
    Natural Environmental Factors
    Technological Factors
        Sociocultural Factors in Reactions to Disasters: The Case of the Exxon *Valdez*
Psychological Factors and Physical Disorders
    Headaches
        Theoretical Perspectives

Narcolepsy
Breathing-Related Sleep Disorder
Circadian Rhythm Sleep Disorder
Parasomnias
Nightmare Disorder
Sleep Terror Disorder
Sleepwalking Disorder
Treatment of Sleep Disorders
Biological Approaches
Psychological Approaches

LEARNING OBJECTIVES

The following learning objectives can also be found at the beginning of the chapter. When you have completed your study of the chapter, you should be able to:

1. Describe the features of adjustment disorders.
2. Explain how labeling an adjustment disorder a "mental disorder" may blur the line between what is normal and what is abnormal.
3. Explain what is meant by a multifactorial view of health and illness.
4. Explain the significance of biological factors in health and illness, paying special attention to the role of the immune system.
5. Explain the significance of psychological factors in health and illness.
6. Explain the significance of socioeconomic, sociocultural, and ethnic factors in health and illness.
7. Explain the significance of natural environmental factors in health and illness.
8. Explain the significance of technological factors in health and illness.
9. Discuss the origins and treatment of headaches.
10. Discuss the origins, risk factors, and treatment of cardiovascular disorders.
11. Discuss the origins and treatment of gastrointestinal disorders.
12. Discuss the origins and treatment of asthma.
13. Discuss the origins and treatment of obesity.
14. Discuss the origins, risk factors, and treatment of cancer.
15. Explain why a discussion of AIDS is included in an abnormal psychology textbook.
16. Discuss the origins and prevention of AIDS.
17. Discuss the diagnostic features of sleep disorders.
18. Discuss the methods of assessment of sleep disorders.
19. Describe the features of the major types of dyssomnias: primary insomnia, primary hypersomnia, narcolepsy, breathing-related sleep disorder, and circadian rhythm sleep disorder.
20. Describe the features of the major types of parasomnias: nightmare disorder, sleep terror disorder, and sleepwalking disorder.
21. Discuss pharmacological and psychological treatments of sleep disorders.

KEY TERMS AND CONCEPTS

The following is a list of terms, concepts, and names that are discussed in the chapter. They are important for you to know. Review these terms, comparing your answers with the material presented in the text.

Rene Descartes
Dualism
Health psychologists
Stress
Stressor
Distress
Adjustment disorders
Immune system
Pathogens
Leukocytes
Antigens
Antibodies
Vaccination
Inflammation
Psychoneuroimmunology
Life changes
Hans Selye
General adaptation syndrome (GAS)
Alarm reaction
Fight-or-flight reaction
Resistance stage
Exhaustion stage
Catecholamines
Emotion-focused coping
Problem-focused coping
Self-efficacy expectancies
Psychological hardiness
Type A behavior pattern
Survivor guilt
Psychosomatic
Psychophysiological
Common migraine
Classic migraine
Individual response specificity
Biofeedback training
Electromyographic
Thermistor
Mediation
Transcendental meditation

Mantras
Progressive relaxation
Edmund Jacobson
Joseph Wolpe
Arnold Lazarus
Cardiovascular disease
Arteriosclerosis
Atherosclerosis
Myocardial infarction
Essential hypertension
Hot reactors
Low-density lipoprotein (LDL) cholesterol
High-density lipoprotein (HDL) cholesterol
Asthma
Obesity
Metabolic rate
Fat cells
Set point
Kelly Brownell
Judith Rodin
Cancer
Human Immunodeficiency Virus (HIV)
Acquired Immunodeficiency Syndrome (AIDS)
Insomnia
Primary insomnia
Sleep disorders
Polysomnographic (PSG) recording
Dyssomnias
Parasomnias
Hypersomnia
Narcolepsy
Cataplexy
REM sleep
Sleep paralysis
Hypnagogic hallucinations
Breathing-related sleep disorder
Obstructive sleep apnea
Circadian rhythm sleep disorder
Nightmare disorder
Sleep terror disorder
Sleepwalking disorder
Hypnotics
Tolerance effect

MATCHING

Match the following names, terms, and concepts with the definitions listed below. The answers are found at the end of the chapter.

a. leukocytes
b. migraine headache
c. cardiovascular disorders
d. distress
e. alarm reaction
f. essential hypertension
g. arteriosclerosis
h. psychosomatic
i. sleep paralysis
j. psychological hardiness
k. cataplexy
l. tension headache
m. survivor guilt

n. psychoneuroimmunology
o. emotion-focused coping
p. pathogens
q. asthma
r. self-efficacy expectation
s. progressive relaxation
t. antibodies
u. dyssomnia
v. individual response specificity
w. fight or flight
x. atherosclerosis
y. immune system
z. problem-focused coping

1) _____ proteins produced by leukocytes that identify and destroy antigens

2) _____ system for recognizing and destroying pathogens that enter our bodies

3) _____ white blood cells that search and destroy pathogens

4) _____ interdisciplinary field concerned with psychological factors and the immune system

5) _____ mobilizes the body for action

6) _____ the body's initial mobilization in response to a stressor

7) _____ a state of physical or mental pain or suffering

8) _____ includes bacteria, viruses, fungi, worn-out body cells, and cells that have become cancerous

9) _____ high levels of commitment, challenge, and perceived control

10) _____ a person's beliefs about their ability to cope or to change

11) _____ negative feelings experienced by those who survive disasters

12) _____ an example of this might be an individual taking measures to immediately reduce the impact of a stressor

13) _____ allergic reaction that constricts bronchi

14) _____ physical disorders in which psychological factors are believed to play a causal or contributing role

15) _____ the idea that people may respond to a stressor in idiosyncratic ways

16) _____ method to increase awareness and control of muscular tension and relaxation

17) _____ intense, piercing pain resulting from changes in blood flow to the brain

18) _____ gradually developing, dull steady pain resulting from stress-induced muscle contraction

19) _____ thickening and hardening of the arteries

20) _____ deposition of fatty substances along walls of arteries

21) _____ examples of this include coronary heart disease, hypertension, and atherosclerosis

22) _____ high blood pressure for which there is no identifiable physical cause

23) _____ an example of this might be an individual examining a stressor and doing what they can to change or modify their own reactions in order to render the stressor less harmful

24) _____ characterized by disturbances in the amount, quality, or timing of sleep

25) _____ a temporary state following awakening in which the person feels incapable of moving or talking

26) _____ a sudden loss of muscular control

TRUE-FALSE

The following true-false statements are reprinted here from your text. Can you remember the answers? They can be found at the end of this chapter.

1. _____ Trouble concentrating on your schoolwork because of the breakup of a recent romance could result in your being labeled as having a "mental disorder."
2. _____ As you read this page, millions of microscopic warriors in your body are engaged in search-and-destroy missions against invading hordes.
3. _____ Stress places people at greater risk for forming dental cavities.
4. _____ Optimistic people recover more rapidly than pessimistic people from coronary artery bypass surgery.
5. _____ A sense of humor may buffer the impact of stress.
6. _____ African Americans are more likely than non-Hispanic, white Americans to die from cancer.
7. _____ Japanese American men who reside in California and Hawaii are more likely than Japanese men who reside in Japan to become obese.
8. _____ People have relieved migraine headaches by raising the temperature in a finger.
9. _____ Dieting has become the normal way of eating for American women.
10. _____ People with insomnia should try harder to make themselves fall asleep.
11. _____ Episodes of sudden, irresistible sleep during the day are actually quite common and raise little concern.
12. _____ Some people literally gasp for breath hundreds of times during sleep without realizing it.

MULTIPLE CHOICE

The multiple choice questions listed below will test your understanding of the material presented in the chapter. Read through each question and circle the letter representing the best answer. The answers are found at the end of the chapter.

1) Which of the following events is less than 30 life-change units (LCUs) on the Holmes and Rahe scale?

    a. marriage
    b. divorce
    c. son or daughter leaving home
    d. pregnancy

2) The correct order of stages in the general adaptation syndrome (GAS) is:

    a. exhaustion, alarm, resistance
    b. alarm, resistance, exhaustion
    c. alarm, exhaustion, resistance
    c. resistance, alarm, exhaustion

3) Which of the following occurs during the alarm stage in the GAS:

    a. muscle tension increases
    b. blood pressure drops
    c. respiration rates decline
    d. epinephrine levels decrease

4) Which of the following is TRUE of leukocytes:

    a. they produce antigens to identify pathogens
    b. they cause inflammation of injured areas
    c. they are foreign invaders in our bodies
    d. they form the basis of the body's immune response

5) Which of the following is NOT considered to be a dyssomnia?

    a. primary hypersomnia
    b. breathing-related sleep disorder
    c. sleepwalking disorder
    d. circadian rhythm sleep disorder

6) Among the mildest of psychological disorders, this is a maladaptive reaction to an identified stressor that develops within a few months of the onset of the stressor.

    a. Major Depressive Episode
    b. Generalized Anxiety Disorder
    c. Panic attacks
    d. Adjustment Disorder

7) Which of the following is the placement of a weakened form of an antigen in the body, which activates the creation of antibodies and memory lymphocytes:

    a. antigens
    b. inflammation
    c. vaccination
    d. antibodies

8) All of the following are true of sleep apnea EXCEPT:

   a. alcohol use before bedtime can be helpful in opening breathing passageways
   b. the disorder is more common in men than in women
   c. when lapses of breathing occurs, the sleeper may suddenly sit up, gasp for
      air, take a few deep breaths, and fall back asleep without awakening
   d. the disorder often goes unnoticed by the afflicted person until it is diagnosed

9) Research shows that stress is:

   a. buffered by social support
   b. unrelated to social support
   c. increased by social support
   d. negatively correlated with social support

10) All of the following are true of a multifactorial view of health and illness EXCEPT:

   a. it provides insight into causation
   b. it suggests multiple pathways of prevention and treatment
   c. it involves psychosocial and medical approaches
   d. it does not take into account biological factors when studying illness

11) All of the following play a role in buffering the effects of stress EXCEPT:

   a. psychological hardiness
   b. optimism
   c. Type A personality
   d. sense of humor

12) Emotion-focused coping includes all of the following EXCEPT:

   a. failure to recognize the seriousness of the problem situation
   b. ignoring the threat of information about the problem situation
   c. denying the threat of the problem situation
   d. all of the above

13) Which of the following adjectives best describes the Type A personality?

   a. highly driven
   b. easy-going
   c. passive
   d. none of the above

14) _____ Americans are nearly one-third more likely to develop hypertension than _____ Americans.

    a. Hispanic; African
    b. Non-hispanic white; Hispanic
    c. Non-hispanic white; African
    d. African; Non-hispanic white

15) Aspirin and ibuprofen relieve pain by:

    a. inhibiting production of prostaglandins
    b. increasing production of prostaglandins
    c. inhibition of serotonin production
    d. inhibition of estradiol production

16) From a biological perspective, essential hypertension is viewed as:

    a. the result of constricted blood vessels due to organic disease
    b. cardiovascular response to pent-up feelings of anger and hostility
    c. the result of the cardiovascular system overreacting to stress
    d. the result of dilated blood vessels due to organic disease

17) REM sleep:

    a. is a period of sleep that occurs after the onset of sleep and involves visual, auditory, tactile, and
       kinesthetic sensations
    b. typically follows several stages of non-REM sleep and is associated with dreaming
    c. typically includes repeated disruptions of sleep due to respiratory problems
    d. involves sleep disruption due to the blockage of air flow in the upper airways

18) Research indicates that _____ may be as prominent a risk factor for CHD as smoking, obesity, and a high fat diet.

    a. divorce
    b. chronic anger
    c. depression
    d. isolation from primary support system

19) All of the following are true of obesity EXCEPT:

    a. the incidence of obesity is highest among the upper socioeconomic status
    b. childhood obesity frequently sets the stage for a chronic course of lifelong obesity
    c. most dieters put almost all of their lost pounds back on within a year
    d. the prevalence of obesity in the United States has doubled since 1900

20) CHD risk can be reduced by:

    a. engaging in anaerobic exercise; aerobic exercise does not decrease risk
    b. the use of emotion-focused coping skills
    c. eating diets high in coconut and palm oils
    d. seeking increased personal control over productivity in the workplace

21) Which of the following is NOT a valuable psychological component in cancer treatment:

    a. prevention of taste aversions
    b. teaching cognitive and behavioral coping skills
    c. use of thermal biofeedback to control pain
    d. use of guided imagery and relaxation training to control nausea

22) All of the following are important roles of mental health professionals in meeting the challenge of the AIDS epidemic EXCEPT:

    a. providing individuals with the means of altering high risk behavior
    b. developing community support for mandatory AIDS testing among high risk populations
    c. counseling homosexual men who engage in high risk sexual behavior
    d. conducting prevention research to find more effective ways to change high risk behaviors

23) Which of the following has become the fastest growing exposure category for HIV infection?

    a. blood transfusion transmission
    b. heterosexual transmission
    c. bisexual transmission
    d. needle-sharing transmission

24) All of the following are true of insomnia EXCEPT:

 a. although the sleep disturbance causes fatigue, it does not affect the
    individual's performance in social, occupational, or other roles
 b. people with primary insomnia have trouble falling asleep or remaining asleep
 c. people with primary insomnia have difficulty achieving restorative sleep
 d. chronic insomnia affects more older people than younger people

25) Which of the following was the 17th century French philosopher who influenced
modern thinking with his belief in dualism:

 a. Rene Descartes
 b. Kelly Brownell
 c. Judith Rodin
 d. Hans Selye

26) Which of the following is characterized by a sleep attack in which the individual
suddenly falls asleep without any warning at various times during the day?

 a. sleep paralysis
 b. obstructive sleep apnea
 c. sleep terror
 d. narcolepsy

27) Which of the following is NOT considered a risk factor for CHD:

 a. ethnicity
 b. gender
 c. age
 d. all of the above are risk factors

28) All of the following are stress-related changes in the body associated with the
alarm reaction stage in the GAS model EXCEPT:

 a. blood coagulability elevates
 b. pupils dilate
 c. sugar is released by the liver
 d. digestion is inhibited

29) Nightmares generally occur during which stage of sleep?

 a. Stage I
 b. Stage II
 c. REM
 d. Stage IV

30) All of the following are problems with using tranquilizers to combat insomnia EXCEPT:

    a. users can become psychologically dependent on the drugs
    b. the drugs have proven to be effective for only approximately half of the people who use them
    c. rebound insomnia can follow discontinuation of the drug
    d. regular use can lead to a "tolerance effect" where progressively larger doses must be used to achieve the same effect

QUESTIONS FOR CRITICAL THINKING

1. Discuss how labeling an adjustment disorder as a mental disorder blur the line between what is normal and what is not.
2. Discuss the current limitations of psychoneuroimmunology.
3. Discuss why it is important to be cautious about interpretations of life change research.
4. Discuss the importance of taking a multifactorial view of health.
5. Compare and contrast emotion-focused coping with problem-focused coping. What are the advantages and disadvantages of each?
6. Discuss the factors that might be helpful in mediating stress among African Americans.
7. Discuss why there were ethnic differences in reaction to the Exxon Valdez disaster.
8. Discuss how individual response specificity explains why only some people get headaches under stress.
9. Discuss some of the reasons why African Americans have high rates of hypertension.
10. Outline a profile of a person with a typical Type A behavior pattern. Can you identify any of these traits in yourself? Do you see these traits as being helpful or harmful to your health? Identify some ways an individual might try to decrease Type A behavior.
11. Discuss how heredity is related to obesity.
12. Discuss how obesity is related to socioeconomic and ethnic factors.
13. Discuss how effective dieting and drugs are in weight loss.
14. Discuss the ideas that the text had on ways to prevent AIDS. Do you agree or disagree with these interventions? Why?
15. Describe the features of the major types of dyssomnias.
16. Describe the features of the major types of parasomnias.
17. Briefly outline and discuss the various treatment approaches for sleep disorders. What are the advantages and disadvantages of these approaches?

ANSWERS FOR MATCHING

1.	t	10.	r	19.	g
2.	y	11.	m	20.	x
3.	a	12.	o	21.	c
4.	n	13.	q	22.	f
5.	e	14.	h	23.	z
6.	w	15.	v	24.	u
7.	d	16.	s	25.	i
8.	p	17.	b	26.	k
9.	j	18.	l		

TRUE-FALSE ANSWERS

1.	T	5.	T	9.	T
2.	T	6.	T	10.	F
3.	T	7.	T	11.	F
4.	T	8.	T	12.	T

MULTIPLE CHOICE ANSWERS

1.	c	11.	c	21.	c
2.	b	12.	d	22.	b
3.	a	13.	a	23.	b
4.	d	14.	d	24.	a
5.	c	15.	a	25.	a
6.	d	16.	c	26.	d
7.	c	17.	b	27.	d
8.	a	18.	b	28.	b
9.	a	19.	a	29.	c
10.	d	20.	d	30.	b

CHAPTER SIX

ANXIETY DISORDERS

OVERVIEW

The <u>name</u> of this family of disorders tells you something important. Each disorder classified here is included because the primary complaint is some form of anxiety, anxiety so extreme that it interferes with the individual's ability to function. The chapter introduces anxiety disorders and their historical perspective, and then describes the following major disorders in this family: panic disorders, generalized anxiety disorders, phobic disorders, obsessive-compulsive disorder, and acute and posttraumatic stress disorders. The major theoretical perspectives on each of these anxiety disorders are described, and the efficacy (effectiveness) of various treatments are evaluated in the discussion of research utilizing specific approaches.

CHAPTER OUTLINE

Historic Perspectives on Anxiety Disorders
    Panic Disorder
    Generalized Anxiety Disorder
    Phobic Disorders
        Specific Phobias
        Social Phobia
        Agoraphobia
    Obsessive-Compulsive Disorder
    Acute and Posttraumatic Stress Disorders
        PTSD among Combat Veterans
            PTSD and the Vietnam Veteran
            Why Vietnam was Worse
Theoretical Perspectives
    Psychodynamic Perspectives
    Learning Perspectives
        The "Value" of Avoiding Fear-Evoking Stimuli
        Reinforcement of Obsessive-Compulsive Behavior
        Prepared Conditioning
        Generalized Anxiety Disorder: A Safety Perspective
        A Conditioning Model of Posttraumatic Stress Disorder
        Observational Learning
    Cognitive Perspectives
        Overprediction of Fear
        Irrational Beliefs
        Oversensitivity to Threats

Low Self-efficacy Expectancies
Self-Defeating Thought
Misattributions for Panic Sensations
Research on Cognitive Factors in Panic Disorders
Biological Perspectives
Genetic Factors
Neurotransmitters
Biological Aspects of Panic Disorder
Sociocultural Factors and Anxiety Disorders
Multiple Pathways in Anxiety Disorders
Treatment of Anxiety Disorders
Psychodynamic Approaches
Humanistic-Existential Approaches
Biological Approaches
Learning-based Approaches
Systematic Desensitization
Gradual Exposure
Cognitive Restructuring
Behavioral Treatment of Social Phobia
Behavioral Treatment of Agoraphobia
Behavioral Treatment of Posttraumatic Stress Disorder
Behavioral Treatment of Obsessive-Compulsive Disorder
Cognitive-Behavioral Treatment of Generalized Anxiety
Rational-Emotive Therapy and Cognitive Therapy
Cognitive-Behavioral Treatment of Panic Disorder

LEARNING OBJECTIVES

The following learning objectives can also be found at the beginning of the chapter. When you have completed your study of the chapter, you should be able to:

1. Describe the chief features of anxiety.
2. Discuss historical changes in the classification of anxiety disorders.
3. Define and describe panic disorder, and explain the differences between panic attacks and other forms of anxiety.
4. Define and describe generalized anxiety disorder.
5. Define and describe specific phobia, social phobia, and agoraphobia.
6. Define and describe obsessive-compulsive disorder.
7. Describe the features of acute and posttraumatic stress disorders.
8. Explain why the Vietnam conflict may have been more likely than others to induce PTSD.
9. Describe various theoretical perspectives on the anxiety disorders.
10. Describe various methods for treating anxiety disorders.
11. Discuss evidence concerning the effectiveness of drug therapies and psychological interventions in treating anxiety disorders.

KEY TERMS AND CONCEPTS

The following is a list of terms, concepts, and names that are discussed in the chapter. They are important for you to know. Review these terms, comparing your answers with the material presented in the text.

Anxiety
Panic disorder
Anxiety disorder
Neuroses
Diagnostic and Statistical Manual of Mental Disorders (DSM)
Psychoses
Generalized anxiety disorder
Phobia
Fear
Specific phobias
Acrophobia
Claustrophobia
Animal type
Natural environment type
Blood-injection-injury type
Situational type
Other type
Social phobia
Agoraphobia
Obsession
Compulsion
Delusions
Acute stress disorder
Posttraumatic stress disorder
Dissociation
Projection
Displacement
O. Hobart Mowrer
Two-factor model
John Watson
Rosalie Rayner
Prepared conditioning
Hyperventilation
Sodium lactate
Neuroticism
Sandra Scarr
Gamma-aminobutyric acid (GABA)
Benzodiazepines
Fear-stimulus hierarchy

Joseph Wolpe
Cognitive restructuring
Exposure therapy
Flooding
Gradual exposure
Stress management skills
Eye movement desensitization and reprocessing (EMDR) treatment
Breathing retraining
David Barlow

MATCHING

Match the following names, terms, and concepts with the definitions listed below. The answers are found at the end of the chapter.

a. gradual exposure
b. systematic desensitization
c. flooding
d. agoraphobia
e. acrophobia
f. neurosis
g. phobias
h. fear
i. compulsion
j. dissociation
k. social phobia
l. sodium lactate
m. anxiety

n. prepared conditioning
o. projection/displacement
p. cognitive restructuring
q. Mowrer's two factor model
r. etiology
s. imipramine
t. acute stress disorder
u. rational-emotive therapy
v. self-defeating thoughts
w. obsession
x. claustrophobia
y. psychosis
z. breathing retraining

1) _____ informal term for severe disorders usually involving loss of contact with reality

2) _____ according to cognitive perspective, these serve to heighten and perpetuate anxiety disorders

3) _____ a treatment approach that has the client maintain a state of calmness in the physical presence of successive stimuli in a fear-stimulus hierarchy

4) _____ recurring, uncontrollable thoughts that create anxiety sufficient to interfere with daily life

5) _____ an antidepressant drug that has produced some positive results with phobia disorders and mixed results with panic disorder

6) _____ cognitive therapy developed by Albert Ellis that shows clients how irrational beliefs contribute to anxiety

7) _____ persistent fears disproportionate to the threat posed by stimuli which elicit them

8) _____ this term is derived from roots meaning "an abnormal or diseased condition of the nervous system"

9) _____ the fear of heights

10) _____ the causes of a disorder; often forms the basis for classification

11) _____ the idea that people may be genetically prepared to acquire phobic responses to certain classes of stimuli

12) _____ the feeling of anxiety and agitation in response to a threat

13) _____ intense, irrational fear of being judged negatively by others

14) _____ induces feelings of panic in some people, especially in people with panic disorder

15) _____ irresistible, repetitive urge to perform a specific action

16) _____ the process therapists use to help clients pinpoint their self-defeating thoughts and generate rational alternatives

17) _____ intense, irrational fear of being out in open, busy areas

18) _____ a treatment in which the client applies counterconditioning to the imagined presence of successive stimuli in a fear-stimulus hierarchy

19) _____ the fear of a neutral object learned through classical conditioning, and maintained through operant avoidance

20) _____ a type of exposure therapy in which the client is exposed to intensely anxiety-provoking situations

21) _____ feelings of detachment from oneself or one's environment

22) _____ generalized fear or apprehension about what might happen

23) _____ a cognitive-behavioral treatment for panic disorder which aims at restoring a normal level of carbon dioxide in the client's blood

24) _____ a psychodynamic defense mechanism for phobias

25) _____ the fear of enclosed spaces

26) _____ stress reaction occurring shortly after a traumatic event

TRUE-FALSE

The following true-false statements are reprinted here from your text. Can you remember the answers? They can be found at the end of this chapter.

1. _____ Some people are suddenly overtaken by feelings of panic and feel they are having a heart attack, even though there is nothing wrong with their heart.
2. _____ Some people live in dread of receiving injections even though the potential pain doesn't bother them a bit.
3. _____ Some people are so fearful of leaving their homes that they cannot even walk down the block to mail a letter.
4. _____ Some people feel compelled to check and recheck that they have locked the doors and windows, so much so that they are delayed in leaving the house for an hour or more.
5. _____ Although we tend to think of posttraumatic stress disorder in terms of the experiences male combat veterans, women are about twice as likely to develop the disorder during their lifetimes than are men.
6. _____ Misinterpretations of minor changes in bodily sensations may be involved in triggering panic attacks.
7. _____ Relaxing in a recliner and fantasizing can be an effective way of reducing fears.
8. _____ You may be able to deter a panic attack by breathing into a paper bag.

MULTIPLE CHOICE

The multiple choice questions listed below will test your understanding of the material presented in the chapter. Read through each question and circle the letter representing the best answer. The answers are found at the end of the chapter.

1) Generalized anxiety is:

    a. more pervasive than panic disorder
    b. more common in men
    c. triggered by situations
    d. never free floating

2) All of the following are explanations of panic disorder EXCEPT:

    a. it is acquired through classical conditioning and maintained by avoidance
    b. it results from intense ego activity to prevent sexual or aggressive impulses from reaching consciousness
    c. it results from catastrophic misinterpretations of body sensations that turn into vicious circles
    d. it is thought to involve serotonin and norepinephrine

3) Obsessive-Compulsive Disorder has been shown to respond best to which drug(s)?

    a. stimulants
    b. tranquilizers
    c. antidepressants
    d. MAO inhibitors

4) The arrangement of stimuli in a sequence as part of systematic desensitization is called:

    a. progressive relaxation
    b. fear stimulus hierarchy
    c. gradual exposure
    d. cognitive orientation

5) According to which theory is anxiety caused by the social repression of our genuine selves?

    a. psychodynamic
    b. cognitive
    c. humanistic-existential
    d. behavioral

6) All of the following are physical features of anxiety EXCEPT:

    a. excessive verbalization
    b. sweaty palms
    c. heavy perspiration
    d. dizziness

7) Most compulsions fall into which two categories?

    a. morning rituals and bedtime rituals
    b. checking rituals and bedtime rituals
    c. bedtime rituals and cleaning rituals
    d. checking rituals and cleaning rituals

8) Vulnerability in experiencing PTSD in response to a traumatic event depends on:

    a. severity of the trauma and degree of exposure
    b. availability of social support
    c. differences in neurobiological responsivity to traumatic experiences
    d. all of the above

9) Which of the following treatments focuses on altering a client's self-defeating thoughts and beliefs:

    a. cognitive approaches
    b. psychodynamic approaches
    c. behavioral approaches
    d. existential-humanistic approaches

10) Which of the following is characterized by persistent and excessive levels of anxiety and worry that is not tied to any particular object, situation, or activity:

    a. agoraphobia
    b. panic disorder without agoraphobia
    c. generalized anxiety disorder
    d. posttraumatic stress disorder

11) Anxiety disorders were classified as neuroses in the first two editions of the DSM. This was largely due to:

    a. William Cullen's assumption that anxiety disorders had underlying biological causes
    b. anxiety disorders being grouped with more serious disturbances
    c. Freud's view that anxiety disorders represented various ways of protecting the ego from anxiety
    d. anxiety disorders being highly resilient to treatment

12) Which of the following factors most likely lessened the incidence of PTSD in Vietnam veterans?

    a. if the veteran was married
    b. if the veteran was divorced
    c. if the veteran lived alone
    d. if the veteran had never married

13) According to the psychodynamic perspective, panic disorder is a result of:

    a. an overprediction of fear, which leads to avoidance
    b. desperate attempts of the ego to repress sexual or aggressive impulses that approach the boundaries of consciousness
    c. a vicious cycle resulting from misinterpretation of bodily sensations
    d. the fear that repressed impulses might become conscious

14) Which of the following is true of Obsessive-Compulsive Disorder?

    a. it affects women more than men
    b. if affect men more than women
    c. it affects women and men in about equal numbers
    d. there is no research on OCD regarding differences in gender

15) Which of the following is the most logical first step in helping a client to develop a fear-stimulus hierarchy to alleviate the fear of riding elevators:

    a. standing outside the elevator
    b. standing in the elevator with the door closed
    c. taking the elevator up one floor
    d. taking the elevator down to the basement

16) This is a new and controversial technique that has emerged in the treatment of PTSD in which the client is asked to picture an image associated with the trauma while the therapist rapidly moves a finger back and forth in front of the client's eyes for approximately 15-20 seconds.

    a. relaxation training
    b. biofeedback
    c. visual image processing (VIP)
    d. eye movement desensitization and reprocessing (EMDR)

17) All of the following are cognitive features of anxiety EXCEPT:

    a. fear of losing control
    b. clear and specific thoughts about the anxiety-inducing situation
    c. keen awareness of bodily sensations
    d. worrying about something

18) Which of the following is NOT a subtype of specific phobias:

    a. Blood-injection-injury type
    b. Generalized type
    c. Animal type
    d. Natural environment type

19) If parents squirm, grimace, or shudder at a spider crawling on the floor, their children:

    a. may learn to respond to spiders with fear and avoidance behavior
    b. will eventually develop panic attacks in response to spiders
    c. will most likely ignore the parents reaction and only develop fears in reaction
       to their own experiences
    d. none of the above

20) Which of the following factors has been shown to be the strongest predictor of suicide attempts and suicidal thoughts by Vietnam veterans:

    a. survivor guilt
    b. depression
    c. anxiety
    d. combat guilt

21) Which of the following are NOT true of panic disorder?

    a. panic disorder is associated with a strong sense of uncontrollability
    b. first attacks typically occur spontaneously or unexpectedly
    c. there are significant phisical differences between cued and uncued panic
       attacks, and it is therefore easy to distinguish them
    d. panic disorder is often associated with agoraphobia

22) In exposure therapy, people with social phobias are instructed to:

    a. enter increasingly stressful social situations and remain in those situations until their urge to escape has lessened
    b. visualize themselves in a stressful social situation and practice relaxation breathing until their anxiety decreases
    c. enter increasingly stressful social situations and remain in those situations until their urge to escape has become too great to stay any longer
    d. identify the stressful components that comprise their anxiety in social situations and work on decreasing the stress associated with these components, one at a time

23) There is a significant amount of research evidence that supports the effectiveness of _____ therapy for panic disorder.

    a. psychodynamic
    b. cognitive-behavioral
    c. existential-humanistic
    d. there is no evidence that one type of treatment is more effective than another

24) Cognitive therapists attribute Obsessive-Compulsive Disorder to:

    a. tendencies to exaggerate the risk of negative outcomes and to adopt irrational beliefs
    b. an irrational concern about broad life themes, such as finances, health, and family matters
    c. hidden, unconscious conflicts
    d. a manifestation of our unmet needs

25) Which of the following is NOT an element of cognitive-behavioral treatment of panic disorder:

    a. self-monitoring
    b. exposure
    c. development of coping responses
    d. insight

26) Which of the following developed systematic desensitization on the assumption that maladaptive anxiety responses are learned or conditioned:

    a. Albert Ellis
    b. Joseph Wolpe
    c. Albert Bandura
    d. John Watson

27) Which of the following is an inhibitory neurotransmitter that regulates nervous activity by preventing neurons from overly exciting their neighbors:

    a. serotonin
    b. norepinephrine
    c. GABA
    d. dopamine

28) In a study conducted by The Epidemiologic Catchment Area (ECA), they found that both African Americans and Hispanic Americans were more likely than their non-Hispanic white counterparts to develop _____ yet were less likely to develop _____.

    a. panic disorder; phobic disorders
    b. phobic disorders; panic disorder
    c. generalized anxiety disorder; PTSD
    d. PTSD; generalized anxiety disorder

29) In treating anxiety disorders, humanistic-existential approaches:

    a. aim at helping people get in touch with and express their genuine talents and feelings
    b. help the client explore sources of anxiety that arise from current relationships
    c. would utilize systematic desensitization in working with the client
    d. help the client to identify and resolve unconscious conflict

30) All of the following are true of using drug therapy to treat panic disorder EXCEPT:

    a. the client may attribute improvement to the drug and not to their own resources
    b. relapses are common following discontinuation of the drugs
    c. it is more effective if cognitive techniques are incorporated with the drug therapy
    d. there have been no problems identified in using drug therapy to treat panic disorder

QUESTIONS FOR CRITICAL THINKING

1.   Discuss why the DSM no longer uses the word "neurosis".
2.   Discuss what we know about anxiety disorders in ethnic minorities.
3.   Compare and contrast panic disorder with agoraphobia and panic disorder without agoraphobia.
4.   Discuss why the Vietnam War was more likely than other wars to induce PTSD.
5.   Compare and contrast specific phobia, social phobia, and agoraphobia.

6. Compare Freud and learning theorists in their explanations of Little Hans.
7. Identify and discuss what are some of the challenges to the behaviorist notions of anxiety disorders.
8. How might PTSD be conditioned?
9. Discuss the role genetics plays in anxiety disorders.
10. Discuss how exposure has been used to treat phobias.
11. Discuss how response prevention may be helpful in treating compulsive behavior.
12. Discuss some of the ways of controlling a panic attack.
13. Compare and contrast psychodynamic, humanistic-existential, biological, and learning-based approaches in the treatment of anxiety disorders.

ANSWERS FOR MATCHING

1.	y	10.	r	19.	q
2.	v	11.	n	20.	c
3.	a	12.	h	21.	j
4.	w	13.	k	22.	m
5.	s	14.	l	23.	z
6.	u	15.	i	24.	o
7.	g	16.	p	25.	x
8.	f	17.	d	26.	t
9.	e	18.	b		

TRUE-FALSE ANSWERS

1.	T	4.	T	7.	T
2.	T	5.	T	8.	T
3.	T	6.	T		

MULTIPLE CHOICE ANSWERS

1.	a	11.	c	21.	c
2.	a	12.	a	22.	a
3.	c	13.	b	23.	b
4.	b	14.	c	24.	a
5.	c	15.	a	25.	d
6.	a	16.	d	26.	b
7.	d	17.	b	27.	c
8.	d	18.	b	28.	b
9.	a	19.	a	29.	a
10.	c	20.	d	30.	d

CHAPTER SEVEN

DISSOCIATIVE AND SOMATOFORM DISORDERS

OVERVIEW

If your previous knowledge of abnormal psychology came from movies and television, then the two types of disorders in this chapter should be very familiar. Although dissociative and somatoform disorders are frequently an important element in movies and television programs, these two disorders are, in fact, rather rare. They are much rarer than most of the other disorders about which you will study.

The Diagnostic and Statistical Manual (DSM) once classified dissociative and somatoform disorders as neuroses. The neuroses consisted of those disorders caused by people's attempt to deal with anxiety. Most contemporary analyses of abnormal behavior still discuss dissociative and somatoform disorders together. Although these two disorders show markedly different symptoms, most theoretical viewpoints agree that avoidance of anxiety underlies both of these disorders.

This chapter first examines dissociative disorders followed by somatoform disorders. As usual, the chapter discusses the major diagnosis criteria for each of the specific disorders included in these broad categories of disorder. This is followed by a discussion of the theories for each disorder and approaches to treatment.

CHAPTER OUTLINE

Dissociative Disorders
    Dissociative Identity Disorder
    Dissociative Amnesia
    Dissociative Fugue
    Depersonalization Disorder
    Theoretical Perspectives
        Psychodynamic Perspectives
        Learning and Cognitive Perspectives
    Treatment of Dissociative Disorders
        Psychodynamic Approaches
        Biological Approaches
        Behavioral Approaches
Somatoform Disorders
    Conversion Disorder
    Hypochondriasis
    Somatization Disorder
    Theoretical Perspectives
    Treatment of Somatoform Disorders
Summary

LEARNING OBJECTIVES

The following learning objectives can also be found at the beginning of the chapter. When you have completed your study of the chapter, you should be able to:

1. Distinguish the dissociative and somatoform disorders from the anxiety disorders in terms of the theorized role of anxiety.
2. Describe the historical changes in the classification of these diagnostic classes.
3. Describe the chief features of the dissociative disorders.
4. Describe dissociative identity disorder.
5. Describe dissociative amnesia and explain how it differs from other types of amnesia.
6. Describe dissociative fugue.
7. Describe depersonalization disorder.
8. Explain why inclusion of depersonalization disorder as a dissociative disorder generates controversy.
9. Discuss problems in differentiating dissociative disorders from malingering.
10. Recount various theoretical perspectives on the dissociative disorders.
11. Explain the theoretical significance of the Spanos study that was inspired by the case of the Hillside strangler.
12. Describe various methods for treating dissociative disorders.
13. Describe the features of conversion disorder, hypochondriasis, and somatization disorder.
14. Discuss theoretical perspectives on somatoform disorders.
15. Distinguish somatoform disorders from malingering.
16. Describe the features of Munchausen syndrome.
17. Discuss theoretical perspectives on Munchausen syndrome.

KEY TERMS AND CONCEPTS

The following is a list of terms, concepts, and names that are discussed in the chapter. They are important for you to know. Review these terms, comparing your answers with the material presented in the text.

Dissociative disorders
Somatoform disorders
Dissociative identity disorder
Dissociative amnesia
Dissociative fugue
Depersonalization disorder
Nicholas Spanos
Derealization
Localized amnesia
Selective amnesia

Generalized amnesia
Continuous amnesia
Systematized amnesia
Malingering
Depersonalization
Repressed memories
Conversion disorder
Hysteria or hysterical neurosis
La belle indifference
Hypochondriasis
Koro syndrome
Dhat syndrome
Somatization disorders
Primary gains
Secondary gains
Munchausen syndrome
Factitious disorders

MATCHING

Match the following names, terms, and concepts with the definitions listed below. The answers are found at the end of the chapter.

a. somatoform disorders
b. hysterical neurosis
c. hypochondriasis
d. selective amnesia
e. Munchausen syndrome
f. dissociative fugue
g. repressed memories
h. derealization
i. conversion disorder
j. dissociative identity disorder
k. somatization disorder
l. localized amnesia
m. systematized amnesia

n. dissociative amnesia
o. la belle indifference
p. dissociative disorders
q. Dhat syndrome
r. depersonalization disorder
s. continuous amnesia
t. factitious disorder
u. primary gain
v. malingering
w. Koro syndrome
x. secondary gain
y. generalized amnesia
z. Nicholas Spanos

1) _____ disorders showing physical symptoms without organic basis or anxiety

2) _____ amnesia for specific details of a stressful event

3) _____ external rewards for symptomatic behavior

4) _____ a former name for conversion disorder, treatment of this illness played a prominent role in the development of psychoanalysis

5) _____ recurrent and multiple physical complaints that usually involve different organ systems in the absence of organic abnormalities

6) _____ disorders showing psychological difficulties without manifest anxiety

7) _____ the fear that genitals are shrinking and retracting into one's body

8) _____ an apparent lack of concern about a conversion disorder symptom

9) _____ a continuing inability to remember events after a trauma

10) _____ an abnormal fear that a physical symptom is due to an underlying serious illness

11) _____ dissociative amnesia with a change of location and a new identity

12) _____ loss of a sensory or motor function without physical cause

13) _____ a sudden loss of memory not attributable to physical problems

14) _____ dissociative amnesia for a fixed period of time following a trauma

15) _____ traumatic memories that have been recovered from the past

16) _____ an inability to remember any of the details of one's life

17) _____ psychodynamic term for relief from unconscious conflicts

18) _____ identity, memory, or consciousness are no longer integrated

19) _____ consciously and deliberately faking symptoms to obtain rewards

20) _____ excessive fears over the loss of seminal fluid during nocturnal emission, often associated with sexual difficulties

21) _____ marked changes in the perception of one's surroundings or time

22) _____ intentional fabrication of symptoms with no apparent goal

23) _____ theorized that multiple personality may result from role-playing to social cues

24) _____ a specific type of factitious disorder when persons tell outrageous lies to physicians and subject themselves to unnecessary medical procedures

25) _____ recurrent feelings of detachment from one's body

26) _____ memories relating to specific categories of information are lost, for example, memories of specific persons in one's life

TRUE-FALSE

The following true-false statements are reprinted here from your text. Can you remember the answers? They can be found at the end of this chapter.

1. _____ Some people have several personalities, and each personality may have its own allergies and eyeglass prescription.
2. _____ People with multiple personality are merely playing a role.
3. _____ Experienced clinicians can determine whether or not people are faking amnesia for their misdeeds.
4. _____ At some time or another, the majority of young adults feel they are detached from their own bodies or thought processes.
5. _____ The great majority of people with multiple personalities were physically or sexually abused as children.
6. _____ College students can be cued to adopt the role of a multiple personality.
7. _____ People have lost all feeling in their hands and legs, although nothing has been medically wrong with them.
8. _____ In China, 2,000 people in the 1980's feel prey to the belief that their genitals were shrinking and retracting into their bodies.
9. _____ Some people show up repeatedly at hospital emergency rooms, feigning illness and seeking treatment for no apparent reason.

MULTIPLE CHOICE

The multiple choice questions listed below will test your understanding of the material presented in the chapter. Read through each question and circle the letter representing the best answer. The answers are found at the end of the chapter.

1) The first two DSM's grouped anxiety, dissociative, and somatoform disorders together because:

    a. the learning perspective assumes that all of these disorders are due to anxiety
    b. the psychodynamic perspective assumes that all of these disorders are due to anxiety
    c. the cognitive perspective assumes that all of these disorders result from a lack of meaning in one's life
    d. the psychodynamic perspective assumes that all of these disorders result from either heterophobia or homophobia

2) Research on dissociative identity disorder suggests that:

    a. the frequency of this disorder is stable across Western countries
    b. the disorder has become less frequent in our culture in the last 20 years
    c. the disorder appears to be culture bound and restricted to North America
    d. the disorder is more prevalent in Japan than North America

3) Which dissociative disorder is most subject to treatment?

    a. depersonalization disorder
    b. dissociative identity disorder
    c. dissociative fugue
    d. dissociative amnesia

4) Diagnosis of a conversion disorder:

    a. requires the presence of multiple physical symptoms
    b. always involves a loss of sexual functioning
    c. is a relatively straightforward diagnosis to make and is not hard to differentiate from medical disorders
    d. should be considered in the case of a false pregnancy

5) Epidemiological research on somatization disorder suggests that:

   a. it is more frequently diagnosed in women
   b. it usually begins in adolescence or early adulthood
   c. it is a lifelong disorder
   d. all of the above

6) According to some learning theorists, hypochondriasis is a form of:

   a. schizophrenia
   b. manic-depressive disorder
   c. dissociative identity disorder
   d. obsessive-compulsive disorder

7) A symptom that may be present in both dissociative identity disorder and schizophrenia is:

   a. split affect
   b. auditory hallucinations
   c. thought disorder
   d. localized amnesia

8) The DSM suggests that the majority of young adults will encounter the feeling that they are detached from their bodies or minds. They are NOT diagnosed as having a depersonalization disorder because:

   a. they are too young to be diagnosed
   b. depersonalization only involves emotions
   c. the detachment is only temporary
   d. young adults are never disturbed by the experience

9) Persons suffering from conversion disorder differ from persons malingering in that persons suffering from a conversion disorder:

   a. are not consciously inventing symptoms
   b. are more likely to be blind
   c. have symptoms with a definite organic basis
   d. receive no secondary gains

10) Nicholas Spanos conducted an experiment modeled after the interrogation of the Hillside strangler, Kenneth Bianchi. Results included which of the following statements?

    a. his control group spontaneously reported a second self 35% of the time
    b. his hidden-part condition refused to answer the Bianchi question
    c. 81% of his Bianchi condition revealed a second self when asked
    d. his subjects who revealed a second self remembered they did so later

11) The individual personalities of a person suffering from a dissociative identity disorder are:

    a. usually schizophrenic
    b. present at the same time
    c. well integrated
    d. always aware of each other

12) Memory should be thought of as:

    a. a reconstructive process in which bits of information are pieced together in a way that is sometimes distorted
    b. a mental camera that stores accurate snapshots of events
    c. an unreliable process that should never be trusted
    d. accurate when objective information is being processed, but less reliable when emotional information is being stored

13) Which feature would NOT be considered a risk factor for the possible presence of dissociative identity disorder?

    a. severe physical or sexual abuse in childhood
    b. a parent with a diagnosis of schizophrenia
    c. suggestibility to hypnotic suggestions
    d. a stormy history of psychological treatment

14) Persons with somatization disorder are more anxious about _____ than are hypochondriacs.

    a. symptoms
    b. problems in interpersonal relationships
    c. failure
    d. memory loss

15) A limitation of the psychodynamic theory of hysteria is:

    a. the theory does not clearly distinguish primary from secondary gain
    b. the theory does not explain how hysterical symptoms are functional
    c. the theory does not explain how energies left over from unconscious conflicts
       become transformed into physical complaints
    d. all of the above

16) Dissociative fugue involves all but one of the following. Which of the following
symptoms is NOT a symptom of a dissociative fugue?

    a. loss of memory for the past
    b. assumption of a new identity
    c. sudden travel from home
    d. a schizophrenic new personality

17) A difference between a malingerer and a person with Munchausen disorder is that:

    a. the malingerer will engage in more dramatic behavior to convince others that
       they are truly ill
    b. the person with Munchausen disorder may be unaware of the underlying
       motives for his or her behavior
    c. the malingerer is more likely to have a childhood history of
       hospitalizations
    d. the person with Munchausen disorder is more likely to 'give up' when
       confronted with evidence of his or her deception

18) According to psychodynamic theory, the process of dissociation is:

    a. an ego-driven processing of fantasy material
    b. a coping mechanism that serves to integrate fantasy and reality
    c. a psychological defense involving a splitting-off of consciousness to block out
       unacceptable memories or impulses
    d. warding off psychological anxiety through the manifestation of physical
       symptoms

19) If a person is unable to remember anything about the week after their father died,
they have what type of dissociative amnesia?

    a. continuous amnesia
    b. generalized amnesia
    c. localized amnesia
    d. selective amnesia

20) Depersonalization disorder differs from the other dissociative disorders in that depersonalization

   a. involves no memory disturbance
   b. produces little distress for the person
   c. symptoms are long lasting
   d. occurs more frequently in females

21) A dissociative fugue state usually ends:

   a. quite suddenly
   b. after shock therapy
   c. after several weeks of taking medication
   d. gradually, over the course of several years

22) Cognitive theorists suggest that the cause of hypochondriasis may stem from:

   a. a cognitive bias to misinterpret emotional cues as physical sensations
   b. a cognitive bias to misinterpret physical sensations as emotional distress
   c. a cognitive bias to misinterpret both physical and emotional symptoms as evidence of psychological disorder
   d. a cognitive bias to misinterpret changes in bodily cues or sensations as signs of catastrophic harm

23) The behavioral approach to treating somatoform disorders may include:

   a. teaching family members to reward attempts to assume responsibility and ignore complaining
   b. focusing on removing sources of secondary reinforcement that may become connected with physical complaints
   c. helping the person learn more effective ways of coping with anxiety
   d. all of the above

24) Which of the following statements about hypochondriasis is TRUE?

   a. it is more frequently diagnosed in women
   b. major depression is rarely diagnosed in individuals with hypochondriasis
   c. people who develop hypochondriasis focus on slight changes in physical status and become anxious about these changes
   d. people who develop hypochondriasis are less likely to have health worries as children

25) An example of a fleeting dissociative experience would be:

    a. feeling dizzy or faint
    b. experiencing chest pains
    c. the feeling that your leg has fallen asleep
    d. finding yourself in a place and not knowing how you got there

QUESTIONS FOR CRITICAL THINKING

1. How is dissociative identity disorder different from schizophrenia?
2. Review the factors that make difficult the diagnosis of dissociative identity disorder.
3. Discuss Kluft's four factor theory of development of dissociative identity disorder.
4. How does amnesia differ from fugue states?
5. What role do traumatic experiences play in dissociative disorders?
6. Where did the term conversion disorder originate?
7. What are Koro and Dhat syndromes?
8. What does it mean to say that hysterical symptoms are functional?
9. What is Munchausen Syndrome by Proxy?

ANSWERS FOR MATCHING

1.	a	10.	c	19.	v	
2.	d	11.	f	20.	q	
3.	x	12.	i	21.	h	
4.	b	13.	n	22.	t	
5.	k	14.	l	23.	z	
6.	p	15.	g	24.	e	
7.	w	16.	y	25.	r	
8.	o	17.	u	26.	m	
9.	s	18.	j			

TRUE-FALSE ANSWERS

1.	T	6.	T
2.	F	7.	T
3.	F	8.	T
4.	T	9.	T
5.	T		

MULTIPLE CHOICE ANSWERS

1.	b	11.	c	21.	a
2.	c	12.	a	22.	d
3.	b	13.	b	23.	d
4.	d	14.	a	24.	c
5.	d	15.	c	25.	d
6.	d	16.	d		
7.	b	17.	b		
8.	c	18.	c		
9.	a	19.	d		
10.	c	20.	a		

CHAPTER EIGHT

MOOD DISORDERS AND SUICIDE

OVERVIEW

This chapter covers mood disorders, including major depression, often referred to as the "common cold" of abnormal psychology. The relatively high frequency of mood disorders makes understanding them important. Because of their prevalence, a great deal of both clinical speculation and research has focused on determining what causes mood disorders and what is the most effective way to treat them. Thus, there are numerous and complex theories and treatments for mood disorders.

The chapter begins with the description of the characteristics of the mood disorders. There are four major mood disorders: major depression, dysthymia, bipolar disorder, and cyclothymia. A discussion of the major theories follows the discussion of the features or diagnostic criteria of the mood disorders. Theories of mood disorders can be grouped into two large categories: the psychological and the biological. Psychodynamic, humanist-existential, learning, and cognitive compose the psychological theories. Genetic and biochemical compose the biological theories. Again, because of the importance of mood disorders, every theoretical perspective tends to more detailed when compared to theories of other disorders you will learn about, with the exception of schizophrenia.

The chapter continues with a discussion of treatments for the mood disorders. These treatments can be grouped in the same way the theories are grouped. The chapter ends with a discussion of suicide and its treatment. Suicide, although not one of the DSM categories, is usually combined with a discussion of depression. This reflects the important association between depression and suicide. An understanding of suicide requires an understanding of depression.

CHAPTER OUTLINE

Mood Disorders
Major Depressive Disorder
      Identified Risk Factors for Major Depression
      Sociocultural Factors in Depression
      Multinational Study of Depression
      Reactive vs. Endogenous Depression
      Seasonal Affective Disorder
      Postpartum Depression
Dysthymic Disorder
Bipolar Disorder
      Manic Episode
Cyclothymic Disorder

LEARNING OBJECTIVES

The following learning objectives can also be found at the beginning of the chapter. When you have completed your study of the chapter, you should be able to:

1. Define mood disorder.
2. Distinguish between normally and abnormally depressed moods.
3. Describe the features of major depressive disorder.
4. Discuss the prevalence of major depressive disorder, with particular attention to ethnic and gender differences and changes in prevalence rates worldwide.

5. Describe the course of major depressive disorder.
6. Discuss seasonal affective disorder.
7. Differentiate between reactive and endogenous depression.
8. Discuss postpartum depression.
9. Differentiate between major depressive disorder, dysthymic disorder, and normal depression.
10. Describe the features of bipolar disorder.
11. Describe the features of a manic episode.
12. Differentiate between bipolar disorder and cyclothymic disorder.
13. Discuss the relationships between stress and mood disorders.
14. Discuss classic and modern psychodynamic perspectives on the mood disorders.
15. Discuss behavioral perspectives on the mood disorders, focusing on the relationships between reinforcement and depression.
16. Discuss cognitive perspectives on depression, focusing on Beck's cognitive theory and the reformulated helplessness (attributional) theory.
17. Discuss genetic factors in the mood disorders.
18. Discuss relationships between biochemical and neuroendocrine factors and mood disorders.
19. Discuss integrative models for understanding depression.
20. Discuss psychodynamic treatment of the mood disorders.
21. Discuss behavioral treatment of the mood disorders.
22. Discuss cognitive treatment of the mood disorders.
23. Discuss the biological treatment of mood disorders.
24. Evaluate the comparative effectiveness of psychotherapy and drug therapy for major depressive disorder.
25. Discuss the incidence of suicide.
26. Discuss theoretical perspectives on the causes of suicide.
27. Discuss methods of suicide prevention.

KEY TERMS AND CONCEPTS

The following is a list of terms, concepts, and names that are discussed in the chapter. They are important for you to know. Review these terms, comparing your answers with the material presented in the text.

Moods
Mood disorders
Unipolar
Bipolar
Major depressive disorder
Manic
Hypomanic
Anhedonia

Bereavement
Psychomotor retardation
Reactive depression
Endogenous depression
Vegetative features of depression
Seasonal affective mood disorder
Postpartum depression
Dysthymia
Double depression
Bipolar I disorder
Bipolar II disorder
Manic episode
Pressured speech
Rapid flight of ideas
Cyclothymia
Hypomanic episode
Mourning
Ambivalent feelings
Introject
Peter Lewinsohn
James Coyne
Aaron Beck
Cognitive triad of depression
Cognitive schemes
Cognitive distortion
Selective abstraction
Catastrophizing
Automatic thoughts
Cognitive-specificity hypothesis
Learned helplessness
Martin Seligman
Attributional style
Internal vs. external attribution
Stable vs. unstable attribution
Global vs. specific attribution
Coping with Depression Course
Catecholamine hypothesis
Tricyclics
MAO inhibitors
Selective serotonin-reuptake inhibitors
Dexamethasone suppression test
Prophylactic
Unilateral vs. Bilateral ECT
Social contagion

MATCHING

Match the following names, terms, and concepts with the definitions listed below. The answers are found at the end of the chapter.

a. bereavement
b. psychodynamic treatment
c. reactive depression
d. interactional theory
e. hypomanic episodes
f. cyclothymia
g. cognitive therapy
h. Peter Lewinsohn
i. mood disorders
j. psychodynamic theory
k. double depression
l. ambivalent
m. human-existential treatment

n. Coping with Depression Course
o. dysthymia
p. reformulated helplessness theory
q. endogenous depression
r. Aaron Beck
s. moods
t. automatic thoughts
u. catecholamine hypothesis
v. postpartum depression
w. anhedonia
x. cognitive-specificity hypothesis
y. human-existential theory
z. tricyclics and monoamine oxidase inhibitors

1) _____ the theory that depression is due to the types of attributions a person makes

2) _____ developed a behavioral theory of depression, emphasizing lack of reinforcement in the environment

3) _____ the theory that different disorders are characterized by different automatic thoughts

4) _____ mild but persistent depressed mood for a period of at least two years

5) _____ habitual thoughts that are accepted without analysis as facts

6) _____ developed a well-known cognitive theory of depression

7) _____ the theory that acting depressed elicits subtle negative reactions from significant others

8) _____ major depression in response to a specific loss

9) _____ treatment of depression which focuses on identifying distorted thoughts and substituting rational ones

10) _____ periods of elevated mood with less severe symptoms and impairment than manic episodes

109

11) _____ the theory that depression is due to a disruption in personality identity due to a loss

12) _____ long periods of mildly elevated or depressed mood

13) _____ serious disturbances in mood that impair day-to-day functioning

14) _____ depression results from deficient levels of norepinephrine

15) _____ major depressive episode superimposed on an episode of dysthymia

16) _____ treatment of depression which focuses on attempts to uncover ambivalent feelings toward lost object

17) _____ persistent depressed mood following childbirth

18) _____ the inability to experience pleasure

19) _____ normal reaction to the death of another person

20) _____ the theory that depression is due to anger turned inward against the self

21) _____ drugs that increase norepinephrine levels in the brain

22) _____ treatment of depression that focuses on finding meaning through self-actualization

23) _____ enduring states of feeling that color our psychological lives

24) _____ simultaneously experienced strongly negative and strongly positive feelings

25) _____ behavioral treatment of depression emphasizing relaxation, pleasant activities, and social skills

26) _____ major depression without any apparent external cause

TRUE-FALSE

The following true-false statements are reprinted here from your text. Can you remember the answers? They can be found at the end of this chapter.

1. _____ It is abnormal to feel depressed.
2. _____ Bleak winter light casts some people into a diagnosable state of depression.

3. ____ Some people ride an emotional roller coaster, swinging from the heights of elation to the depths of depression without external cause.

4. ____ In some ways, many "mentally healthy" people see things LESS realistically than people who are depressed.

5. ____ Prozac is the most widely used antidepressant in the United States, even though it is known to prompt suicidal behavior.

6. ____ The ancient Greeks and Romans used a contemporary form of chemotherapy to treat turbulent mood swings.

7. ____ Suicide is a sign of insanity.

8. ____ People who threaten to commit suicide are only seeking attention.

MULTIPLE CHOICE

The multiple choice questions listed below will test your understanding of the material presented in the chapter. Read through each question and circle the letter representing the best answer. The answers are found at the end of the chapter.

1) Which of the following would be typical of a normally depressed person?

    a. depressed mood passes quickly
    b. large decrease in physical activity
    c. recurrent thoughts of suicide
    d. faulty perceptions of reality

2) Which of the following is a diagnostic feature of major depression?

    a. short periods of depressed mood
    b. deliberate increase in weight
    c. persistent inability to sleep
    c. repetitive and stereotyped motoric activity

3) Interpersonal therapy for depression differs from traditional psychodynamic treatments in that:

    a. interpersonal therapy focuses on the clients' current relationships
    b. interpersonal therapy focuses on early childhood experiences
    c. interpersonal therapy focuses on conflicts between the ego and the superego
    d. interpersonal therapy focuses on establishing goals for the future

4) If you think you are dealing with a person who is considering committing suicide, which of the following statements would be the best response?

    a. "You're talking crazy."
    b. "Let's wait and see how you feel next week."
    c. "Come with me and we'll find some help."
    d. "You're just being silly."

5) A person who overcomes an episode of major depression:

    a. is unlikely to have another one within a two year period
    b. has a 50% chance of having one in two years
    c. is more likely to have another episode the longer they go on without one
    d. is more likely to develop a psychotic disorder than a person who has never had an episode

6) The three types of attributions most vulnerable to depression are:

    a. external, global, and unstable attributions
    b. external, specific, and unstable attributions
    c. internal, specific, and stable attributions
    d. internal, global, and stable attributions

7) Which theory of suicide suggests and emphasizes that people committing suicide do so because they believe that it will solve their problems?

    a. psychoanalytic
    b. social-learning
    c. interpersonal
    d. existential-humanist

8) Among which age group are suicide rates the highest?

    a. young children
    b. adolescents
    c. mature adults
    d. the elderly

9) Which of the following groups has the highest rate of depression?

    a. women who have never been married
    b. married men
    c. married women
    d. men who have recently been divorced

10) The tendency to "make mountains out of molehills" is referred to as:

    a. catastrophizing
    b. mental filtering
    c. overgeneralizing
    d. musterbation

11) Lithium as a treatment of bipolar disorder:

    a. is extremely safe with few side effects
    b. has clearly understood pharmacological effects
    c. can be discontinued once normal mood is established
    d. is the most widely used drug for treatment of manic episodes

12) Which of the following is one way that dysthymia differs from major depression?

    a. major depression lasts longer than dysthymia
    b. dysthymia is characterized by mild hypomanic episodes
    c. major depression functions as part of a person's personality
    d. dysthymia's mood alteration is less severe

13) Low motivation and energy, feelings of sadness, suicidal ideation, psychomotor retardation, and apathy are features of which kind of depression?

    a. reactive depression
    b. hopelessness depression
    c. interpersonal depression
    d. seasonal depression

14) Major depression affects how many adults?

    a. approximately one in one hundred
    b. nearly one in twenty
    c. nearly one in five
    d. almost one-half of the adult population

15) MAO inhibitors:

    a. block the activity of an enzyme
    b. stimulate release of neurotransmitters
    c. inhibit reuptake sites on postsynaptic membranes
    d. are safer to take than tricyclics

16) Bipolar disorder is characterized by:

   a. one or two years of mania followed by a year or two of depression
   b. short manic episodes followed by longer depressive episodes
   c. short depressive episodes followed by longer manic episodes
   d. four or five manic-depressive cycles per year

17) Research on the self-focusing model of depression suggests that:

   a. depressed persons typically do not focus on themselves but on other people
   b. depressed persons focus on themselves more than others following successes
   c. self-focused attention has been linked to disorders other than depression
   d. self-focused attention in depressed people is lower following failures

18) Which of the following is NOT one of the characteristics of a manic episode?

   a. pressured speech
   b. psychomotor retardation
   c. rapid flight of ideas
   d. impaired social judgment

19) Learning theory suggests that inactivity and depressed feeling of a depressive episode usually produces:

   a. little change in the environment, which maintains a stable level of depression
   b. little response by one's family and thus acting out for attention
   c. a further decrease in reinforcement and increasingly severe depression
   d. sympathy and understanding from one's family resulting in less severe depression

20) Cognitive therapy seeks to help clients recognize cognitive distortions. Which of the following is an example of a cognitive distortion?

   a. "I know I'm going to flunk this course."
   b. "Stop blaming yourself for everyone else's problems."
   c. "Feeling something doesn't make it so."
   d. "Nobody is destined to be a loser."

21) Which of the following may act as a buffer against the onset of depression during stressful times?

   a. social support
   b. being wealthy
   c. living in the same city as one's parents
   d. having the same job for several years

22) MZ twins show _____ concordance for major depression and _____ concordance for bipolar disorder than DZ twins:

   a. higher; higher
   b. higher; lower
   c. lower; lower
   d. lower; higher

23) Which of following types of delusions would be most likely to be found in depression?

   a. delusions of persecution ("Somebody is out to get me")
   b. delusions of grandeur ("I am the reincarnation of Buddha")
   c. delusions of reference ("The book on display with the title 'Making Your Will' is a message that I am going to die this week")
   d. delusions of unworthiness or guilt ("I have committed a terrible crime")

24) Psychodynamic theories of depression focus on _____, learning theories emphasize _____.

   a. intrapsychic determinants of disorders; cultural factors
   b. cognitive determinants of disorders; interpersonal factors
   c. inner, sometimes unconscious determinants of disorders; situational factors
   d. interpersonal determinants of disorders; cognitive factors

25) According to psychoanalytic theory, the _____ is the dominant part of the personality during depressive episodes of bipolar disorder.

   a. conscious
   b. id
   c. ego
   d. superego

26) Which is NOT considered a risk factor for depression?

    a. living in an urban area
    b. socioeconomic status
    c. educational level
    d. marital status

27) People who experience a repeated pattern of severe fall and winter depression may be diagnosed with:

    a. endogenous depression
    b. seasonal affective disorder
    c. cyclothymia
    d. vegetative depression

28) Which of the following is NOT part of the cognitive triad of depression?

    a. negative beliefs about oneself
    b. negative beliefs about the environment
    c. negative beliefs about the past
    d. negative beliefs about the future

29) In the dexamethasone test for depression, depression is indicated by:

    a. high levels of cortisol
    b. low levels of cortisol
    c. low levels of dexamethasone
    d. high levels of epinephrine

30) Which of the following treatments have been shown to be effective for the treatment of depression, according to the guidelines issued by an expert panel in 1993?

    a. antidepressant medication
    b. cognitive therapy, behavior therapy, and interpersonal therapy
    c. other specified treatments such as ECT
    d. all of the above

QUESTIONS FOR CRITICAL THINKING

1.   Why is depression termed the common cold of psychological problems?
2.   What factors might explain gender differences in depression?
3.   What are some limitations of the reactive-endogenous depression distinction?
4.   Describe what is meant by "rapid cycling".

5. Contrast the self-focusing model with traditional psychodynamic theory.
6. Review the empirical support for Lewinsohn's model of depression.
7. What are the differences between the original and revised learned helplessness model for depression? What does the revised version account for that the original version did not?
8. What are the weaknesses of the dexamethasone suppression test as a diagnostic indicator for depression?
9. Compare and contrast interpersonal psychotherapy with traditional psychodynamic approaches.
10. What are the advantages of prescribing an antidepressant such as Prozac to a depressed person? What are the limitations of antidepressant medications?
11. Pretend that you are treating a client who is currently hospitalized for severe depression. Would you recommend ECT? What factors would influence your decision?
12. Compare the psychodynamic, cognitive, and social learning theories of suicide. Which theory do you think best explains suicide? Why?

ANSWERS FOR MATCHING

1.	p	10.	e	19.	a
2.	h	11.	y	20.	j
3.	x	12.	f	21.	z
4.	o	13.	i	22.	m
5.	t	14.	u	23.	s
6.	r	15.	k	24.	l
7.	d	16.	b	25.	n
8.	c	17.	v	26.	q
9.	g	18.	w		

TRUE-FALSE ANSWERS

1.	F	5.	F
2.	T	6.	T
3.	T	7.	F
4.	T	8.	F

MULTIPLE CHOICE ANSWERS

1.	a	11.	d	21.	a
2.	c	12.	d	22.	a
3.	a	13.	b	23.	d
4.	c	14.	c	24.	c
5.	b	15.	c	25.	d
6.	d	16.	b	26.	c
7.	b	17.	c	27.	b
8.	d	18.	b	28.	c
9.	c	19.	c	29.	a
10.	a	20.	a	30.	d

CHAPTER NINE

PERSONALITY DISORDERS

OVERVIEW

In learning about the classification of abnormal behavior back in Chapter 3, you learned that personality disorders were classified on Axis II of DSM. This chapter considers those personality disorders. You will learn the defining features of personality disorders--the things they have in common that serve to separate them from other behavior disorders. Personality disorders are divided into three clusters based on types of behavior. You will learn about these three clusters and the specific personality disorders that fall within them. Consideration of the personality disorders is not complete without a discussion of the problems in their classification. Theoretical perspectives and treatment of personality disorders are very brief sections. If you have been progressing through the text section by section, you should find the section on theoretical perspectives to be straightforward and relatively easy. Personality disorders are viewed as very resistant to change, making treatment a difficult task. In the treatment section the authors of the text give you information to help you develop a real appreciation for therapists' views of what they are up against.

CHAPTER OUTLINE

Personality Disorders
      Types of Personality Disorders
Personality Disorders Characterized by Odd or Eccentric Behavior
      Paranoid Personality Disorder
      Schizoid Personality Disorder
      Schizotypal Personality Disorder
Personality Disorders Characterized by Dramatic, Emotional, or Erratic Behavior
      Antisocial Personality Disorder
            Historical Perspectives on Antisocial Personality Disorder
            Sociocultural Factors and Antisocial Personality Disorder
            Antisocial Behavior and Criminality
            Profile of Antisocial Personality Disorder
      Borderline Personality Disorder
      Histrionic Personality Disorder
      Narcissistic Personality Disorder
Personality Disorders Characterized by Anxious or Fearful Behavior
      Avoidant Personality Disorder
      Dependent Personality Disorder
      Obsessive-Compulsive Personality Disorder
Problems with the Classification of Personality Disorders
      Undetermined Reliability and Validity

LEARNING OBJECTIVES

The following learning objectives can also be found at the beginning of the chapter.
When you have completed your study of the chapter, you should be able to:

1. Define personality disorder.
2. Discuss controversies in diagnosing personality disorders.
3. Describe the features of paranoid, schizoid, and schizotypal personality
    disorders.
4. Describe the features of antisocial, borderline, histrionic, and narcissistic
    personality disorders.
5. Describe the features of avoidant, dependent, and obsessive-compulsive
    personality disorders.
6. Discuss problems in the classification of personality disorders, including their
    reliability and validity, and sexist biases.
7. Discuss theoretical perspectives on the personality disorders.
8. Discuss the special problems in treating personality disorders.

KEY TERMS AND CONCEPTS

The following is a list of terms, concepts, and names that are discussed in the chapter. They are important for you to know. Review these terms, comparing your answers with the material presented in the text.

Personality disorders
Ego-syntonic
Ego-dystonic
Paranoid personality disorder
Schizoid personality disorder
Schizotypal personality disorder
Simple schizophrenia
Ideas of reference
Antisocial personality disorder
Psychopath
Sociopath
Phillipe Pinel
J. R. Prichard
Hervey Cleckley
Perseveration
Borderline personality disorder
Histrionic personality disorder
Narcissistic personality disorder
Avoidant personality disorder
Dependent personality disorder
Obsessive-compulsive personality disorder
Hans Kohut
Self psychology
Otto Kernberg
Splitting
Margaret Mahler
Symbiosis
Separation-individuation
Theodore Millon
Ullmann and Krasner
Albert Bandura
Problem-solving therapy
Galvanic skin response
Optimum level of arousal
Cerebral cortex
Limbic system
Dialectical behavior therapy
Token economies

MATCHING

Match the following names, terms, and concepts with the definitions listed below. The answers are found at the end of the chapter.

a. ego-dystonic
b. sociopath
c. dialectical behavior therapy
d. optimum level of arousal
e. splitting
f. Ullmann and Krasner
g. simple schizophrenia
h. emotional responsiveness
i. personality disorders
j. cerebral cortex
k. cluster B: dramatic or erratic
l. Achievement Place
m. separation-individuation

n. J. R. Prichard
o. Otto Kernberg
p. limbic system
q. ideas of reference
r. ego-syntonic
s. cluster A: odd or eccentric
t. "healthful narcissism"
u. symbiosis
v. Hans Kohut
w. galvanic skin response
x. cluster C: anxious or fearful
y. Hervey Cleckley
z. Margaret Mahler

1) _____ biological view that antisocial personality disorder results from lack of anticipatory anxiety

2) _____ excessively rigid patterns of behavior, or ways of relating to others

3) _____ paranoid, schizoid, and schizotypal personality disorders

4) _____ perception that behavior and one's feelings are a natural part of one's self

5) _____ psychodynamic theorist(s) who related narcissistic personality disorder to lack of parental empathy and support

6) _____ an English psychiatrist who conceptualized antisocial personality as "moral insanity"

7) _____ antisocial, borderline, histrionic, and narcissistic personality disorders

8) _____ perception that feelings and behavior are foreign to one's self- identity

9) _____ a degree of arousal at which people feel best and function most efficiently

10) _____ the process of developing a separate psychological and biological identity from the mother and recognizing the defining characteristics of one's own identity

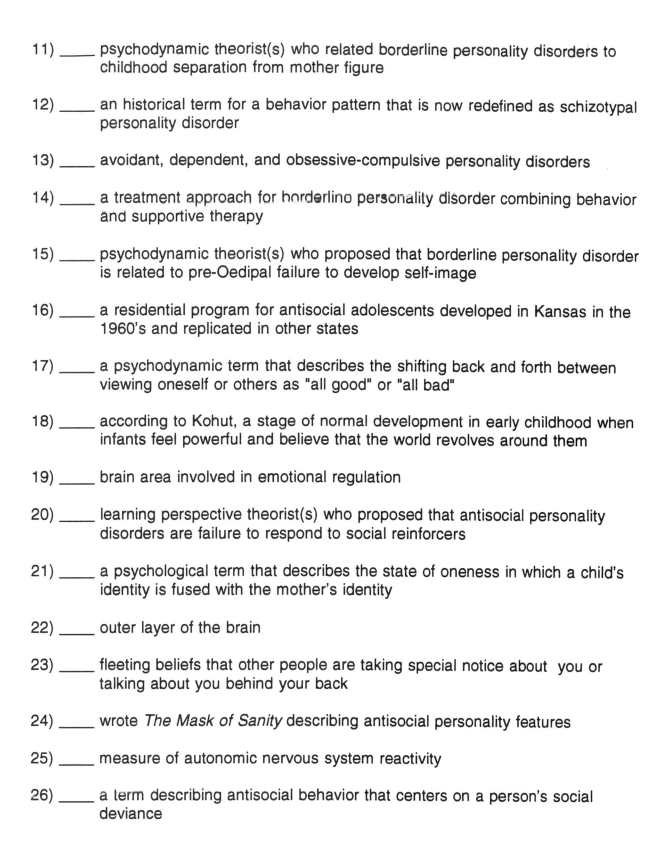

11) _____ psychodynamic theorist(s) who related borderline personality disorders to childhood separation from mother figure

12) _____ an historical term for a behavior pattern that is now redefined as schizotypal personality disorder

13) _____ avoidant, dependent, and obsessive-compulsive personality disorders

14) _____ a treatment approach for borderline personality disorder combining behavior and supportive therapy

15) _____ psychodynamic theorist(s) who proposed that borderline personality disorder is related to pre-Oedipal failure to develop self-image

16) _____ a residential program for antisocial adolescents developed in Kansas in the 1960's and replicated in other states

17) _____ a psychodynamic term that describes the shifting back and forth between viewing oneself or others as "all good" or "all bad"

18) _____ according to Kohut, a stage of normal development in early childhood when infants feel powerful and believe that the world revolves around them

19) _____ brain area involved in emotional regulation

20) _____ learning perspective theorist(s) who proposed that antisocial personality disorders are failure to respond to social reinforcers

21) _____ a psychological term that describes the state of oneness in which a child's identity is fused with the mother's identity

22) _____ outer layer of the brain

23) _____ fleeting beliefs that other people are taking special notice about you or talking about you behind your back

24) _____ wrote *The Mask of Sanity* describing antisocial personality features

25) _____ measure of autonomic nervous system reactivity

26) _____ a term describing antisocial behavior that centers on a person's social deviance

123

TRUE-FALSE

The following true-false statements are reprinted here from your text. Can you remember the answers? They can be found at the end of this chapter.

1. _____ Some people have deeper feelings for animals than they do for people.
2. _____ Some people can intentionally injure others without experiencing feelings of guilt or remorse.
3. _____ It can be difficult to draw the line between normal variations in behavior and personality disorders.
4. _____ The concept of certain types of personality disorders may be sexist.
5. _____ People who have exaggerated views of their own importance may actually harbor deep feelings of inadequacy.
6. _____ People with antisocial personalities tend to remain unduly calm in the face of impending pain.

MULTIPLE CHOICE

The multiple choice questions listed below will test your understanding of the material presented in the chapter. Read through each question and circle the letter representing the best answer. The answers are found at the end of the chapter.

1) Extreme focus on details, rigidity in relationships, limited ability to express feelings, and difficulty relaxing and having fun are characteristic of:

      a. schizoid personality disorder
      b. obsessive-compulsive personality disorder
      c. dependent personality disorder
      d. borderline personality disorder

2) Analogy: fear of rejection is to lack of interest in social relations as:

      a. dependent personality disorder is to schizotypal personality disorder
      b. schizotypal personality disorder is to avoidant personality disorder
      c. avoidant personality disorder is to schizoid personality disorder
      d. schizoid personality disorder is to avoidant personality disorder

3) The term "borderline" was originally used to describe:

   a. people whose behaviors appeared to border between sane and insane
   b. people whose behaviors appeared to border between schizophrenic and manic
   c. people whose behaviors appeared to border between neurotic and psychotic
   d. people whose behaviors appeared to border between depressed and antisocial

4) Which is NOT found in studies of antisocial personality?

   a. ability to learn from experience
   b. high sensation seeking
   c. underresponsive nervous system
   d. brain abnormalities

5) Problem-solving therapy for antisocial adolescent boys may be characterized as:

   a. learning prosocial behaviors to replace antisocial ones
   b. developing self-esteem through making new friends
   c. learning to view antisocial behavior as problematic and not in one's best interests
   d. reconceptualizing social interactions as problems to be solved

6) Which personality disorder name derives from Latin for actor?

   a. histrionic
   b. narcissistic
   c. schizoid
   d. paranoid

7) Research supports the view that people with antisocial personalities:

   a. are more aroused during both rest times and times of stress
   b. are generally less aroused during both rest times and times of stress
   c. are less aroused during times of rest but overreact during stress
   d. are aroused at about the same level as other people both during times of rest and at times of stress

8) Antisocial personality disorder is more common among:

   a. Hispanic Americans
   b. people from lower SES levels
   c. African-Americans
   d. people with childhood psychiatric problems

9) Which of the following is NOT a major controversy in the classification of personality disorders?

    a. too many cases that fit two or more diagnostic categories
    b. excessive ambiguity in diagnostic criteria
    c. inclusion of traits that are normal in lesser degree as key diagnostic criteria
    d. debate as to whether personality disorders need a separate axis in DSM or should be included in Axis I

10) Which of the following statements is true regarding treatment of personality disorders?

    a. people with personality disorders do not usually seek treatment on their own
    b. people with personality disorders often drop out of treatment prematurely
    c. people who seek treatment for disorders such as depression and who also have personality disorders often respond poorly to treatment
    d. all of the above

11) Narcissistic personality disorder is most known for:

    a. disregard for the law
    b. uncertain values
    c. inflated sense of self
    d. social isolation

12) Phillipe Pinel, the French reformer who called for more humane treatment of the mentally ill, introduced what form of therapy?

    a. outdoor therapy
    b. conformity therapy
    c. social therapy
    d. moral therapy

13) About _____ people with personality disorders meet diagnostic criteria for more than one personality disorder.

    a. 1 in 10
    b. 1 in 4
    c. 2 in 3
    d. 1 in 2

14) A commonality of learning theory and psychodynamic theory in explaining the development of personality disorders is:

   a. genetic history of the individual
   b. physical abnormalities present at birth
   c. the person's ability to develop a strong sense of identity
   d. salient childhood experiences

15) For persons under the age of 18, an appropriate diagnosis to consider for antisocial behavior would be:

   a. antisocial personality disorder
   b. schizoid personality disorder
   c. conduct disorder
   d. adjustment disorder

16) Failure to develop a coherent self image is a key sign of:

   a. antisocial personality disorder
   b. borderline personality disorder
   c. histrionic personality disorder
   d. narcissistic personality disorder

17) In which personality disorder does the person find it difficult to do things on his or her own?

   a. dependent
   b. avoidant
   c. obsessive-compulsive
   d. antisocial

18) Which of the following is NOT an example of self-defeating narcissism?

   a. responding to life's wounds with depression or fury
   b. feeling entitled to special treatment and becoming very upset when treated in an ordinary manner
   c. being temporarily wounded by criticism
   d. needing constant support from other people in order to feel good about oneself

19) The concept of self theory has been used most to explain what personality disorder?

   a. narcissistic
   b. antisocial
   c. dependent
   d. histrionic

20) Which of the following personality disorders is more commonly diagnosed in females?

   a. antisocial personality disorder
   b. schizoid personality disorder
   c. paranoid personality disorder
   d. borderline personality disorder

21) Which of these is NOT part of Cleckley's clinical profile of antisocial personality disorder?

   a. responding to setbacks with depression or fury
   b. lack of remorse or shame
   c. inability to profit from experience
   d. superficial charm and intelligence

22) An individual with which personality disorder would be most likely to use splitting?

   a. narcissistic
   b. dependant
   c. avoidant
   d. borderline

23) Beth's behavior is self-destructive. Beth has a borderline personality disorder. Beth's behavior is self-destructive because she has a borderline personality disorder. These statement reflect which kind of faulty reasoning which may be used to validate diagnoses?

   a. concrete reasoning
   b. illogical reasoning
   c. circular reasoning
   d. clinical reasoning

24) Which personality disorder seems to be a caricature of the feminine personality?

    a. histrionic
    b. avoidant
    c. obsessive-compulsive
    d. schizoid

25) People who may appear to be guarded or suspicious might be:

    a. diagnosed with schizoid personality disorder
    b. experiencing ego-dystonic symptoms
    c. unfamiliar with the customs and rules of the majority culture
    d. planning to commit a crime

26) A treatment approach which has NOT been found effective with personality disorders is:

    a. behavior therapy
    b. drug therapy
    c. brief structured psychodynamic therapy
    d. all of the above

QUESTIONS FOR CRITICAL THINKING

1.   How do personality disorders differ from normal styles of behavior?
2.   Compare and contrast the behavior of schizotypal and schizoid personality disordered individuals.
3.   Contrast the terms psychopath and sociopath.
4.   How is antisocial behavior related to criminality?
5.   Why is borderline personality concept close to that of the mood disorders?
6.   How does normal self interest compare with narcissism?
7.   In what ways to personality disorders overlap?
8.   Describe how some personality disorders show a sexist bias.
9.   What does it mean to confuse labels with explanations?
10.   Review the controversial aspects of psychodynamic theories of personality disorders.
11.   Discuss the evidence that support the role of family factors in the development of personality disorders.
12.   What role do genetics play in personality disorders?
13.   Discuss the behavioral treatment approaches to personality disorders.

ANSWERS FOR MATCHING

1.	h	10.	m	19.	p
2.	i	11.	z	20.	f
3.	s	12.	g	21.	u
4.	r	13.	x	22.	j
5.	v	14.	c	23.	q
6.	n	15.	o	24.	y
7.	k	16.	l	25.	w
8.	a	17.	e	26.	b
9.	d	18.	t		

TRUE-FALSE ANSWERS

1.	T	4.	T
2.	T	5.	T
3.	T	6.	T

MULTIPLE CHOICE ANSWERS

1.	b	11.	c	21.	a
2.	c	12.	d	22.	d
3.	c	13.	c	23.	c
4.	a	14.	d	24.	a
5.	d	15.	c	25.	c
6.	a	16.	b	26.	b
7.	b	17.	a		
8.	b	18.	c		
9.	b	19.	a		
10.	d	20.	d		

CHAPTER TEN

SUBSTANCE ABUSE AND DEPENDENCE

OVERVIEW

This chapter explains the relationship of the use of psychoactive chemicals (drugs) and abnormal psychology. It begins by discussing the classification of substance-related disorders and moves into identifying and discussing drugs that are grouped together by pharmaceutical categories such as Depressants, Stimulants, and Hallucinogens. It will be helpful for you to learn to associate specific drugs with the category name to which each belongs. This will help you learn the effects of these drugs, as categories generally have effects in common (although routes of chemical action of specific drugs within a category may differ). It would also be helpful for you to be thoroughly familiar with the major effects of each of the drugs included in the chapter.

The last sections in the chapter deal with theoretical perspectives and treatments of substance abuse. In these sections, more so than the corresponding sections of earlier chapters, you will find considerable controversy. Different theoretical perspectives have led to treatment goals and strategies that are not just different, but may be strongly opposed to one another on specific treatment issues. Similar to the chapter on personality disorders, drug abuse is not easily treated. Some of the reasons for the difficulty of treatment are the same as those outlined in the personality disorder chapter; however, others are specific to the effects of the abused substance.

CHAPTER OUTLINE

Classification of Substance-related Disorders
    Substance Abuse and Dependence
        Who's Most at Risk?
    Addiction, Physiological Dependence, and Psychological Dependence
    Pathways to Drug Dependence
    Intoxication
    Withdrawal Syndromes
        Gateway Drugs
Depressants
    Alcohol
        Alcoholism and Alcohol Use Disorders
        Risk Factors for Alcoholism
        Alcoholism: Disease, Moral Defect, or Behavior Pattern?
        Psychological Effects of Alcohol
        Physical Health and Alcohol
        Moderate Drinking: Is There a Health Benefit?
    Sedatives, Hypnotics, and Antianxiety Drugs

Behavioral Approaches
        Self-control Strategies
        Aversive Conditioning
        Social Skills Training
    Relapse-prevention Training
Summary

LEARNING OBJECTIVES

The following learning objectives can also be found at the beginning of the chapter. When you have completed your study of the chapter, you should be able to:

1. Define substance abuse, substance dependence, substance intoxication, and substance withdrawal.
2. Distinguish between psychological and physiological dependence.
3. Describe U.S. drinking patterns.
4. Discuss risk factors for alcoholism.
5. Discuss the effects of alcoholism.
6. Discuss the effects of sedatives and minor tranquilizers.
7. Discuss the effects of opioids.
8. Discuss the effects of amphetamines.
9. Discuss the effects of cocaine.
10. Discuss the effects of nicotine and tobacco smoke.
11. Discuss the effects of PCP.
12. Discuss the effects of LCD.
13. Discuss the effects of marijuana.
14. Discuss the biological, psychodynamic, learning, cognitive, and sociocultural approaches to substance abuse and dependence.
15. Discuss the biological and behavioral approaches to explaining drug cravings.
16. Discuss the disease model of substance abuse and dependence.
17. Discuss genetic factors in alcoholism.
18. Discuss drug therapy approaches to treatment of substance abuse and dependence.
19. Discuss lay approaches to treatment, such as AA.
20. Discuss behavioral approaches to treatment.
21. Discuss cognitive approaches to treatment.
22. Discuss the need for, and methods of, relapse-prevention training.
23. Discuss the controversial concerning controlled social drinking programs.
24. Discuss problems in evaluating the effectiveness of treatment programs.

KEY TERMS AND CONCEPTS

The following is a list of terms, concepts, and names that are discussed in the chapter. They are important for you to know. Review these terms, comparing your answers with the material presented in the text.

Psychoactive
Substance use disorders
Substance-induced disorders
Substance intoxication
Delirium
Psychotic disorders
Substance abuse
Substance dependence
Withdrawal syndrome
Abstinence syndrome
Addiction
Physiological dependence
Psychological dependence
Pathological gambling
Impulse-control disorder
Kleptomania
Intoxication
Tachycardia
Delirium tremens
Disorientation
Gateway drugs
Depressant
Ethyl alcohol/ethanol
Alcoholism
Antisocial personality disorder
Fetal alcohol syndrome (FAS)
E. M. Jellinek
GABA
Alcoholic hepatitis
Cirrhosis
Alcohol-induced persisting amnestic disorder (Korsakoff's syndrome)
Barbiturates/sedatives
Opioids/narcotics
Analgesia
Endorphins
Morphine
Heroin
Stimulants
Amphetamines

Amphetamine psychosis
Cocaine
John Styth Pemberton
Crack
Freebasing
Cocaine psychosis
Passive smoking
Nicotine
Hemoglobin
Hydrocarbons
Hallucinogens/psychedelics
Lysergic acid diethylamide (LSD)
Flashbacks
Phencyclidine (PCP)/"angel dust"
Deliriant
Marijuana
Delta-9-tetrahydrocannabinol (THC)
Hashish
Negative reinforcement
Cue exposure training
Aaron Beck
Absolutist thinking
Relapse
Mentally ill chemical abuser ("MICA")
Detoxification
Disulfiram (Antabuse)
Desipramine
Nicotine replacement therapy
Methadone
Naloxone
Naltrexone
Alcoholics Anonymous (AA)
Narcotics Anonymous
Cocaine Anonymous
Al-Anon
Synanon
Aversive conditioning
Covert sensitization
Rapid smoking
Controlled social drinking
Relapse-prevention training
Abstinence violation effect (AVE)

MATCHING

Match the following names, terms, and concepts with the definitions listed below. The answers are found at the end of the chapter.

a. freebasing
b. methadone
c. LSD
d. tachycardia
e. endorphins
f. detoxification
g. amphetamines
h. tolerance
i. Al-Anon
j. addiction
k. hashish
l. heroin
m. withdrawal

n. intoxication
o. substance abuse
p. barbiturates
q. Korsakoff's syndrome
r. self-control strategies
s. minor tranquilizers
t. delirium
u. relapse prevention training
v. amphetamine psychosis
w. cirrhosis of the liver
x. stimulants
y. nicotine chewing gum
z. fetal alcohol syndrome

1) _____ continued use of a substance despite knowledge that use is causing the individual to suffer from physical, psychological, social, or occupational problems.

2) _____ a spin-off of AA, this was designed to provide support for families of alcoholics

3) _____ a class of psychoactive substances that increase nervous system activity

4) _____ the process of helping a physiologically dependent individual through the abstinence syndrome

5) _____ neurotransmitters chemically similar to opiate drugs, which are thought to be involved in pleasure and pain experiences

6) _____ a psychoactive substance derived from the resin of a marijuana plant

7) _____ stimulants initially used to extend vigilance, the common abuse pattern is an extended high followed by a "crash" period of deep sleep and/or depression

8) _____ mental confusion and disorientation combined with inability to focus attention

9) _____ a slow-acting opiate used in the treatment of heroin addiction

10) _____ chronic alcohol use causes a protein deficiency, which results in this

11) _____ the process of heating cocaine powder with ether to release its psychoactive chemical base, which is then inhaled

12) _____ with continued use of a substance, higher doses are needed to maintain the same effect

13) _____ a drug that produces visual hallucinations by decreasing serotonin action and increasing dopamine activity

14) _____ a drug-induced state which mimics paranoid schizophrenia

15) _____ includes valium and librium and are known to produce psychological dependence

16) _____ teaching clients how to prevent lapses from resulting in a return to substance dependence

17) _____ a pattern of retarded development and features, this is estimated to affect at least 40% of children born to mothers who drink during pregnancy

18) _____ a grouping of therapies which focus on the ABCs of substance abuse

19) _____ everyday term for habitual use of a drug accompanied by signs of physiological dependence

20) _____ depressant drugs used medically to alleviate anxiety and insomnia

21) _____ behavior changes induced by chemical actions of psychoactive substances

22) _____ a dramatic reduction in the intake of an abused substance, this produces symptoms characteristic of the specific substance on which the individual is physiologically dependent

23) _____ an alcohol induced vitamin B deficiency which produces confusion, disorientation, and memory loss

24) _____ an abnormally rapid heart rate, a component of the effects of alcohol withdrawal

25) _____ a review of placebo-control studies supports its use in combination with behavior therapy to help people stop smoking

26) _____ a drug that was first developed in 1875 to cure morphine addiction

TRUE-FALSE

The following true-false statements are reprinted here from your text. Can you remember the answers? They can be found at the end of this chapter.

1. _____ Legal substances cause more deaths through sickness and accidents than all illicit drugs combined.
2. _____ The use of heroin is rising rapidly on America's campuses.
3. _____ Cocaine is the most widely abused substance in the United States today.
4. _____ You cannot develop a dependence on a drug without becoming addicted.
5. _____ More teenagers die as a result of suicide than any other cause.
6. _____ Alcohol goes to women's heads more rapidly than to men's.
7. _____ Heroin was developed during a search for a drug that would relieve pain as effectively as morphine, but without causing physical addiction.
8. _____ Cigarettes are habit forming but not physically addictive.
9. _____ Being able to "hold your liquor" better than most people may put you at risk of developing a drinking problem.
10. _____ African Americans have higher rates of alcohol abuse and dependence than non-Hispanic white Americans.

MULTIPLE CHOICE

The multiple choice questions listed below will test your understanding of the material presented in the chapter. Read through each question and circle the letter representing the best answer. The answers are found at the end of the chapter.

1) All of the following are examples of substance abuse EXCEPT:

a. repeatedly driving while intoxicated
b. losing sales due to using cocaine prior to a sales presentation with six major clients
c. missing work 13 days in the last six weeks due to alcohol use
d. smoking marijuana at a friend's house on Saturday nights off and on over the past year

2) Which of the following is NOT a diagnostic criteria for psychoactive substance dependence:

a. inability to reduce drug use
b. experiencing intoxication with smaller amounts of the psychoactive substance
c. spending increased time obtaining, using, and recovering from substance use
d. use of the substance to prevent withdrawal symptoms

3) Which of the following is NOT one of the principle patterns of chronic alcohol abuse?

    a. periods of binge drinking separated by long periods of abstinence
    b. regular consumption of large quantities of alcohol
    c. heavy weekend drinking
    d. all of the above are patterns of chronic alcohol abuse

4) Which of the following is true of barbiturates?

    a. quickly produce both physiological and psychological dependence
    b. produce only psychological dependence
    c. produce only physiological dependence
    d. produce neither physiological nor psychological dependence

5) Risk factors for alcoholism include:

    a. sex, age, social class, race, and antisocial personality disorder
    b. age, social class, alcoholism in the family, mood disorders, and obsessive compulsive personality disorder
    c. alcoholism in the family, race, depression, and tobacco use
    d. tobacco use, race, social class, sex, and borderline personality disorder

6) Fetal alcohol syndrome:

    a. requires that the mother drink alcohol only during the third trimester of pregnancy
    b. includes symptoms of narrowly spaced eyes, dwarfism, and mental retardation
    c. affects all children born to mothers who drink alcohol during pregnancy
    d. can occur when the mother drinks only one or two ounces of alcohol per day during pregnancy

7) Which of the following are true of amphetamines?

    a. produce amphetamine psychosis in moderate doses
    b. do not produce tolerance
    c. quickly produce psychological dependence in those who take them to relieve depression
    d. produce neither physiological nor psychological dependence

8) The incidence of heroin abuse:

    a. has declined due to the risk of HIV from the use of unsterile needles
    b. has remained constant since 1975, probably due to the popularity of cocaine and crack cocaine
    c. is largely confined to younger individuals
    d. has increased dramatically, probably due to it being easy to obtain

9) Repeated high-dosage cocaine use:

    a. is nearly always fatal
    b. can result in anxiety and depression
    c. raises the threshold of grand-mal seizures
    d. produces a reverse-tolerance effect

10) The psychedelic drug most likely to induce violent or aggressive behavior is:

    a. LSD
    b. PCP
    c. THC
    d. hashish

11) Delirium and psychotic disorders may be induced during states of intoxication from use of _____ or _____.

    a. alcohol; cocaine
    b. alcohol; nicotine
    c. cocaine; nicotine
    d. cocaine; caffeine

12) All of the following are diagnostic features of substance dependence EXCEPT:

    a. tolerance for the substance
    b. diminished activity in important social, occupational, or recreational activities due to substance use
    c. lack of withdrawal symptoms
    d. continued substance use despite evidence of persistent or recurrent psychological or physical problems associated with its use

13) Tobacco smoke contains which of the following:

    a. THC and nicotine
    b. chlorinated hydrocarbons and carbon monoxide
    c. chlorinated hydrocarbons and nicotine
    d. nicotine and carbon monoxide

14) Which of the following is the most abused substance in the United States:

   a. alcohol
   b. marijuana
   c. cocaine
   d. both alcohol and marijuana

15) Alcoholics Anonymous has adopted many of the ideas and concepts of
_____ in its program.

   a. E.J. Watson
   b. E.M. Jellinek
   c. Aaron Beck
   d. Karen Horney

16) Which of the following is considered an impulse-control disorder?

   a. depression
   b. alcoholism
   c. pathological gambling
   d. weekend drinking binges

17) In psychodynamic theory, alcoholism reflects the role of:

   a. culture
   b. oral dependent personality
   c. self awareness
   d. negative reinforcement

18) Which of the following is TRUE of controlled drinking strategies?

   a. work best with individuals who can abstain from alcohol
   b. help only those with patterns of heavy binge drinking
   c. helpful only for individuals who have gone through withdrawal symptoms
      during detoxification
   d. may be effective with younger drinkers and for those rejecting total
      abstinence

19) _____ is a potentially fatal liver condition in which healthy liver cells become
supplanted with scar tissue.

   a. clrrhosis
   b. Korsakoff's syndrome
   c. alcoholic hepatitis
   d. Crohn's disease

20) LSD is a psychedelic that produces visual hallucinations by _____ the action of _____.

 a. increasing; dopamine
 b. decreasing; dopamine
 c. increasing; serotonin
 d. decreasing; serotonin

21) Which of the following is the tendency to overreact to a lapse?

 a. covert sensitization
 b. relapse stigmatization
 c. abstinence violation effect (AVE)
 d. none of the above

22) _____ and _____ have the highest incidence of alcoholism in the U.S.

 a. Native Americans; Irish Americans
 b. Hispanic Americans; Native Americans
 c. Asian Americans; Irish Americans
 d. Hispanic Americans; Asian Americans

23) In order to be effective in helping people stop smoking, nicotine chewing gum:

 a. must become a permanent substitute for tobacco
 b. must be combined with other forms of treatment
 c. must be prescribed only by a physician
 d. should be used only when the client's craving for a cigarette is low

24) Which of the following is NOT a behavioral treatment for substance abuse?

 a. self-control strategies
 b. aversive conditioning
 c. abstinence violation training
 d. skills training

25) All of the following are opioids EXCEPT:

 a. morphine
 b. heroin
 c. codeine
 d. PCP

26) All of the following are true of depressants EXCEPT:

    a. impairs cognitive processes
    b. increases central nervous system activity
    c. in high doses, can arrest vital functions and cause death
    d. reduces feelings of tension and anxiety

27) Modeling explains, in part, why:

    a. children of alcoholics drink
    b. self efficacy is low in drinkers
    c. tension reduction occurs
    d. genetic factors affect drinking

28) Sigmund Freud was a prominent early advocate of this drug:

    a. heroin
    b. morphine
    c. cocaine
    d. opium

29) Which of the following is NOT considered to be a withdrawal symptom of nicotine:

    a. depressed mood
    b. vomiting
    c. insomnia
    d. tremors

30) High success rates claimed by AA have been criticized on all of the following grounds EXCEPT:

    a. measures of success limited to self-report
    b. up to 90% of the individuals who drop out of AA after a few meetings are not counted in determining success rates
    c. failure to include success rates of control groups
    d. failure to protect anonymity of clients in statistical studies of success

QUESTIONS FOR CRITICAL THINKING

1.   Discuss the effects that legal substance abuse has had on our country.
2.   Compare and contrast substance abuse and substance dependence.
3.   Define "gateway drugs" and describe what they do.
4.   Discuss how alcohol abuse is related to ethnic membership.
5.   Describe the patterns of alcohol use in college students.

6. Identify some ways to determine an alcohol dependency.
7. Describe the disease model of alcoholism and discuss why it is debated.
8. Briefly discuss the effects of the following drugs: amphetamines, cocaine, nicotine, LSD, PCP, and marijuana.
9. Review the history of cocaine use.
10. Identify the possible medical complications of cocaine use.
11. Briefly compare and contrast the biological, psychodynamic, learning, cognitive, and sociocultural approaches to substance abuse and dependence.
12. Explain how genetic factors might contribute to alcoholism.
13. Discuss the limits of nicotine replacement therapy.
14. Discuss the controlled social drinking controversy.
15. Discuss how relapse prevention training differs from the disease model of alcoholism.

ANSWERS FOR MATCHING

1.	o	10.	w	19.	j
2.	i	11.	a	20.	p
3.	x	12.	h	21.	n
4.	f	13.	c	22.	m
5.	e	14.	v	23.	q
6.	k	15.	s	24.	d
7.	g	16.	u	25.	y
8.	t	17.	z	26.	l
9.	b	18.	r		

TRUE-FALSE ANSWERS

1.	T	4.	F	7.	T
2.	F	5.	F	8.	F
3.	F	6.	T	9.	T
				10.	F

MULTIPLE CHOICE ANSWERS

1.	d	11.	a	21.	c
2.	b	12.	c	22.	a
3.	d	13.	d	23.	b
4.	a	14.	a	24.	c
5.	a	15.	b	25.	d
6.	d	16.	c	26.	b
7.	c	17.	b	27.	a
8.	b	18.	d	28.	c
9.	b	19.	a	29.	b
10.	b	20.	d	30.	d

CHAPTER ELEVEN

GENDER IDENTITY DISORDER, ATYPICAL PATTERNS OF SEXUAL BEHAVIOR, AND SEXUAL DYSFUNCTION

OVERVIEW

In order to understand abnormal sexual behavior, one must first consider what is normal. This chapter discusses cultural differences in what sexual behaviors are considered normal and abnormal, and how American culture has changed its views on sexual behavior since World War II. With this perspective, the authors then go on to consider a series of sexual disorders. Something to keep in mind while reading this chapter is that the viewpoint presented is that of a professional psychologist. As a reader, you may either agree or disagree with the perspective of what is considered normal and abnormal in relation to sexuality; however, what is outlined in your text is consistent with the diagnostic guidelines of the DSM-IV. In addition to identifying various sexual disorders, the chapter also includes information such as diagnostic features of the disorder, its incidence, theoretical perspectives, and the efficacy of various treatment methods in working with certain types of sexual dysfunction.

CHAPTER OUTLINE

Normal and Abnormal in Sexual Behavior
Gender and Identity Disorder
    Gender Reassignment Surgery
        Postoperative Adjustment
        Theoretical Perspectives
Paraphilias
    Exhibitionism
    Fetishism
    Transvestic Fetishism
    Voyeurism
    Frotteurism
    Pedophilia
    Sexual Masochism
    Sexual Sadism
    Other Paraphilias
    Theoretical Perspectives
    Treatment of Paraphilias
Sexual Dysfunctions
    The Sexual Response Cycle
    Types of Sexual Dysfunctions
        Sexual Desire Disorders
        Sexual Arousal Disorders

LEARNING OBJECTIVES

The following learning objectives can also be found at the beginning of the chapter.
When you have completed your study of the chapter, you should be able to:

1. Describe sociocultural factors in conceptions of what sexual behaviors are normal and abnormal.
2. Discuss the changes in the DSM concerning the classification of homosexuality as a mental disorder.
3. Describe gender identity disorder.
4. Describe the process of gender reassignment and discuss its success.
5. Define and describe the features of various paraphilias.
6. Discuss theoretical perspectives on the paraphilias.
7. Discuss treatment of persons with paraphilias.
8. Describe the phases of the sexual response cycle.
9. Define and describe the features of various sexual dysfunctions.
10. Discuss theoretical perspectives on sexual dysfunctions.
11. Discuss treatment of the sexual dysfunctions.

KEY TERMS AND CONCEPTS

The following is a list of terms, concepts, and names that are discussed in the chapter. They are important for you to know. Review these terms, comparing your answers with the material presented in the text.

Gender identity disorder
Transsexualism
Gonads
Homosexuality
Ego-dystonic homosexuality
Paraphilias
Exhibitionism
Fetishism
Transvestic fetishism
Voyeurism
Frotteurism
Pedophilia
Sexual masochism
Hypoxyphilia
Sexual sadism
Sadomasochism
Lifelong dysfunctions
Sexual dysfunctions
Acquired dysfunctions
Situational dysfunctions
Generalized dysfunction
William Masters
Virginia Johnson
Helen Singer Kaplan
Appetitive phase
Excitement phase
Orgasm phase
Resolution phase
Hypoactive sexual desire disorder
Sexual aversion disorder
Female sexual arousal disorder
Male erectile disorder/sexual impotence
Female orgasmic disorder
Male orgasmic disorder
Premature ejaculation
Dyspareunia
Vaginismus
Nocturnal penile tumescence (NPT)
Penile strain gauge

Plethysmograph
Albert Ellis
Barlow model
Performance anxiety
Bibliotherapy
Sensate focus exercises
Self-spectatoring
Squeeze technique
Stop-start technique
Papaverine

MATCHING

Match the following names, terms, and concepts with the definitions listed below. The answers are found at the end of the chapter.

a. fetishism
b. dyspareunia
c. voyeurism
d. orgasm phase
e. transsexualism
f. sexual dysfunctions
g. pedophilia
h. sexual impotence
i. Kinsey
j. plethysmograph
k. exhibitionism
l. paraphilia
m. bisexuals

n. Masters & Johnson
o. appetitive phase
p. gender identity
q. sensate focus exercises
r. frotteurism
s. sexual masochism
t. performance anxiety
u. ego-dystonic homosexual
v. excitement phase
w. gender identity disorder
x. transvestic fetishism
y. sexual sadism
z. hypoxyphilia

1) _____ respond sexually to both males and females

2) _____ sexual urges and arousal focused on making a victim suffer humiliation or physical pain

3) _____ published research on sexual normality in the 1960's that fed the fires of the sexual revolution of the 1960's and 1970's

4) _____ conflict between biological gender and gender identity

5) _____ the peak and release of sexual tension

6) _____ presence of sexual fantasies and the desire to engage in sexual activity

7) _____ recurrent urges and fantasies regarding sexual activity with pre-pubescent children

8) _____ sexual arousal to inanimate objects such as clothing

9) _____ persistent feelings of being trapped inside a body with the wrong biological sex

10) _____ Masters & Johnson's therapeutic technique to counter performance anxiety

11) _____ sexual arousal by oxygen deprivation

12) _____ zoologist who published the first scientific surveys of American sexual behavior in the late 1940's and early 1950's

13) _____ involves erection in men and vaginal lubrication in women

14) _____ the psychological sense of being male or female

15) _____ refers to homosexuals who reject their sexual orientation

16) _____ sexual urges and related fantasies involving cross-dressing

17) _____ fear over ability to perform successfully sexually

18) _____ in women, pain in the genital region associated with sexual intercourse

19) _____ a tampon-shaped probe that is placed in the vagina to measure vaginal blood engorgement

20) _____ sexual urges, arousal and fantasy centered on rubbing against or touching a nonconsenting person

21) _____ in men, persistent or recurrent problems in becoming genitally aroused

22) _____ sexual urges and arousal focused on being humiliated or made to physically suffer

23) _____ involve problems with sexual interest, arousal, or response

24) _____ sexual arousal to stimuli that are unusual or bizarre

25) _____ the recurrent, powerful urge to expose one's genitals to an unsuspecting stranger in order to surprise, shock, or sexually arouse the victim

26) _____ watching unsuspecting people who are undressed, disrobing or engaging in sexual activity in order to attain sexual excitement

TRUE-FALSE

The following true-false statements are reprinted here from your text. Can you remember the answers? They can be found at the end of this chapter.

1. _____ Gay males and lesbians suffer from a psychological disorder that involves the desire to become a member of the opposite gender.
2. _____ Homosexuality is a type of mental disorder.
3. _____ Wearing revealing bathing suits is a form of exhibitionism.
4. _____ Watching your sexual partner disrobe is a form of voyeurism.
5. _____ Some people cannot become sexually aroused unless they are subjected to pain or humiliation by others.
6. _____ Orgasm is a reflex.
7. _____ Sexual dysfunctions are rare.
8. _____ Penile implants can help men with erectile dysfunction achieve erections.

MULTIPLE CHOICE

The multiple choice questions listed below will test your understanding of the material presented in the chapter. Read through each question and circle the letter representing the best answer. The answers are found at the end of the chapter.

1) Sexual behaviors are considered disorders when:

a. they are harmful to others
b. they are statistically uncommon in the individual's culture
c. the individual experiences personal distress associated with the behavior
d. all of the above

2) Professional stripteasers and swimmers in revealing bathing suits:

a. meet the clinical criteria for exhibitionism
b. do not meet the clinical criteria for exhibitionism because they are not attempting to sexually arouse the victim
c. do not meet the clinical criteria for exhibitionism because the individuals they are exposing themselves to are not unsuspecting
d. meet the clinical criteria for transvestic fetishism

3) A disorder involving involuntary spasm in the muscles of the vagina which makes sexual intercourse difficult or impossible is:

   a. vaginismus
   b. dyspareunia
   c. female sexual arousal disorder
   d. sexual aversion disorder

4) An example of a mild form of this may be striking one's partner with a feather brush.

   a. transvestic fetishism
   b. sadomasochism
   c. hypoxyphilia
   d. sexual masochism

5) Approximately _____ times as many boys as girls have gender identity disorder.

   a. 2
   b. 3
   c. 5
   d. 10

6) An individual who experiences sexual arousal to members of the same sex:

   a. are diagnosed ego dystonic homosexual only if they accept their sexual orientation
   b. are diagnosed bisexual
   c. are diagnosed ego dystonic homosexual only if they reject their sexual orientation
   d. none of the above

7) The view that paraphilias are the result of some object or activity inadvertently becoming associated with sexual arousal, gaining the ability to elicit that arousal when the individual fantasizes about or acts out the paraphilias, is associated with the _____ perspective.

   a. psychodynamic
   b. learning
   c. cognitive
   d. sociocultural

8) Sexual aversion disorder and hypoactive sexual desire disorder are both:

   a. sexual desire disorders
   b. sexual arousal disorders
   c. orgasm disorders
   d. sexual pain disorders

9) There are some promising results reported in using which medication to treat voyeurism and fetishism?

   a. imipramine
   b. desipramine
   c. prozac
   d. haldol

10) A review of international studies reported positive results from gender reassignment surgery in about:

   a. 25% of cases
   b. 50% of cases
   c. 75% of cases
   d. 90% of cases

11) Sexual reflexes in the excitement and orgasm stages:

   a. occur in women but not in men
   b. occur in men but not in women
   c. are evidence of sexual dysfunction
   d. cannot be willed or forced

12) Psychodynamic theorists view gender identity disorder as the result of:

   a. overly permissive parents
   b. close mother-son relationships combined with empty father-son relationships
   c. close father-son relationships combined with empty mother-son relationships
   d. overly restrictive parents

13) Freud viewed premature ejaculation as symbolic of:

   a. oral fixations
   b. attachment to the father
   c. hatred of women
   d. the electra complex

14) The term "Ego-dystonic homosexuality":

    a. remains a diagnostic category in the DSM-IV
    b. was reclassified as "Sexual disorder not otherwise specified" in the DSM-IV
    c. was reclassified as "Homosexuality" in the DSM-IV
    d. was deleted from the DSM-IV and not reclassified as another disorder

15) Transvestic fetishism is reported:

    a. only among heterosexual men
    b. only among homosexual men
    c. only among heterosexual men and women
    d. only among homosexual men and women

16) Which of the following is quite commonplace and therefore may not be considered abnormal from the statistical perspective?

    a. frotteurism
    b. paraphilias
    c. sexual dysfunctions
    d. all of the above are considered abnormal from the statistical perspective

17) Behavioral and cognitive therapies for paraphilias attempt to:

    a. help the client to accept his/her behavior and fantasies
    b. help the client adapt his/her behavior to minimize the effect it has on others
    c. protect society from these individuals
    d. disconnect arousal from the paraphiliac stimulus and reattach it to normal stimuli

18) Psychological adjustment to sex reassignment:

    a. is more favorable for female-to-male changes
    b. is more favorable for male-to-female changes
    c. has been shown to be poor regardless of direction of change
    d. has been shown to depend upon the quality of the surgical construction of sexual organs

19) All of the following are considered common features of sexual dysfunctions EXCEPT:

    a. emotional effects
    b. assumption of a performer role rather than a spectator role
    c. diminished self-esteem
    d. fear of failure

20) A classic study on adjustment and gay lifestyles conducted by Bell and Weinberg (1978) concluded that:

    a. gay males were more poorly adjusted than heterosexuals
    b. gay males were better adjusted than heterosexuals
    c. gay males in close stable relationships were as well-adjusted as married heterosexuals
    d. none of the above

21) Which of the following paraphilias is relatively harmless and victimless?

    a. pedophilia
    b. exhibitionism
    c. sadism
    d. fetishism

22) Biological factors may account for _____ of erectile dysfunction cases.

    a. 10-19%
    b. 40-50%
    c. 80-90%
    d. virtually all

23) Nocturnal penile tumescence (NPT) refers to:

    a. a device used to monitor time changes in penile erections
    b. a technique used in gender reassignment surgery
    c. a physiological measure to evaluate erections during sleep
    d. none of the above

24) Which of the following is an example of transvestic fetishism?

    a. a heterosexual male who cross-dresses in private and imagines himself to be a woman who he is stroking as he masturbates
    b. a homosexual male who cross-dresses to attract other men
    c. a male with a gender identity disorder who cross-dresses because of gender discomfort associated with wearing men's clothing
    d. all of the above

25) Which of the following theorists proposed a model of erectile dysfunction that takes into account cognitive factors?

   a. Ellis
   b. Barlow
   c. Kaplan
   d. Johnson

QUESTIONS FOR CRITICAL THINKING

1. Discuss what makes sexual behavior abnormal.
2. Identify and discuss the role that biological factors play in sexual orientation.
3. Discuss how the DSM-IV differs from prior DSM's in classifying gender identity disorders.
4. Identify how sexual problems are assessed.
5. Discuss the possible role that anxiety plays with sexual performance.
6. Discuss the efficacy of sex therapy.
7. Discuss how biological approaches may help to treat male erectile disorder.
8. Compare and contrast the following paraphilias: exhibitionism, fetishism, transvestic fetishism, voyeurism, frotteurism, and pedophilia.
9. Compare and contrast sexual sadism with sexual masochism.
10. Discuss the treatment of paraphilias. What are the success rates?
11. Compare and contrast the following types of sexual dysfunction: sexual desire disorders, sexual arousal disorders, orgasm disorders, and sexual pain disorders. What are some of the common features?
12. Identify and discuss the sexual response cycle pioneered by William Masters and Virginia Johnson.
13. Compare and contrast the sex therapy approaches of Masters and Johnson to that of Helen Singer Kaplan.

ANSWERS FOR MATCHING

1.	m	10.	q	19.	j
2.	y	11.	z	20.	r
3.	n	12.	i	21.	h
4.	w	13.	v	22.	s
5.	d	14.	p	23.	f
6.	o	15.	u	24.	l
7.	g	16.	x	25.	k
8.	a	17.	t	26.	c
9.	e	18.	b		

TRUE-FALSE ANSWERS

1.	F	4.	F	7.	F
2.	F	5.	T	8.	T
3.	F	6.	T		

MULTIPLE CHOICE ANSWERS

1.	d	11.	d	21.	d
2.	c	12.	b	22.	b
3.	a	13.	c	23.	c
4.	b	14.	b	24.	a
5.	c	15.	a	25.	b
6.	c	16.	c		
7.	b	17.	d		
8.	a	18.	a		
9.	c	19.	b		
10.	d	20.	c		

CHAPTER TWELVE

SCHIZOPHRENIA AND OTHER PSYCHOTIC DISORDERS

OVERVIEW

This chapter focuses on a disorder that afflicts between one and two percent of the world's population and is responsible for about half of the psychiatric hospitalizations. It will be a challenging chapter for you because it contains a large number of new terms and concepts, all of which are necessary to give you a complete understanding of this very complicated disorder. The unique combination of frequency and severity have made schizophrenia a heavily studied disorder. Yet schizophrenia's complexity has kept it more than a bit of a mystery.

Your chapter opens with a brief history of the disorder, tracing the roots of its discovery and diagnosis by Emil Kraepelin. You will learn about the disorder as perceived by other early theorists such as Eugen Bleuler and Kurt Schneider. Next, your chapter examines how schizophrenia differs from other psychoses and hallucinatory based disorders.

The next section reviews the diagnostic features of schizophrenia, describing these features in detail. A section on the types or sub-classifications recognized under DSM follows. Although they are not recognized under DSM IV, your chapter discusses three additional dimensions of schizophrenia, which are under consideration by researchers.

As with previous chapters, sections discussing theories and therapies of the disorder follow. Each of the major theories of abnormal behavior discussed in chapter two of your text have had a lot to say about both the theory and treatment of schizophrenia. Therefore, the sections on the "Theoretical Perspectives" and "Treatment" of schizophrenia are among the most detailed in the text.

The chapter finishes with a short section on delusional disorder. Delusional disorder is included in this chapter because of the similarity of its symptoms to paranoid schizophrenia.

CHAPTER OUTLINE

History of the Concept of Schizophrenia
      Emil Kraepelin
      Eugen Bleuler
      Kurt Schneider
      Contemporary Diagnostic Practices
Prevalence of Schizophrenia
Phases of Schizophrenia
      Briefer Forms of Psychosis
Schizophrenia-Spectrum Disorders

Family Intervention Programs
Delusional Disorders
Summary

LEARNING OBJECTIVES

The following learning objectives can also be found at the beginning of the chapter. When you have completed your study of the chapter, you should be able to:

1. Discuss the contributions of Emil Kraepelin, Eugen Bleuler, and Kurt Schneider to the concept of schizophrenia.
2. Discuss the changes in the definition of schizophrenia that have occurred from the time of Kraepelin to the present day.
3. Discuss the prevalence of schizophrenia in the general population.
4. Describe the various patterns of the course of schizophrenia, referring to the concepts of acute episode, prodromal phase, and residual phase.
5. Distinguish among schizophrenia, brief psychotic disorder, and schizophreniform disorder.
6. Discuss the concept of schizophrenia-spectrum disorders and distinguish among schizophrenia, schizotypal personality disorder, and schizoaffective disorder.
7. Discuss the disturbances in thought and speech that characterize schizophrenia.
8. Discuss deficits in attention, referring to recent psychophysiological research.
9. Discuss perceptual disturbances in schizophrenia.
10. Discuss emotional disturbances in schizophrenia.
11. Discuss the disturbances in self-identity, volition, interpersonal behavior, and psychomotor behavior in schizophrenia.
12. Discuss the historical changes in the classification of types of schizophrenia.
13. Distinguish between the disorganized, catatonic, paranoid, undifferentiated, and residual types of schizophrenia.
14. Discuss the process-reactive dimension of schizophrenia, the positive and negative symptoms of schizophrenia, and Type I and Type II schizophrenia.
15. Discuss psychodynamic, learning, biological, family, and sociocultural perspectives on schizophrenia.
16. Describe and evaluate research on genetic factors, biochemical factors, viral infections, and brain damage.
17. Discuss evidence for the diathesis-stress model of schizophrenia.
18. Discuss biological, psychoanalytic, learning-based, psychosocial-rehabilitation, and family intervention treatments of schizophrenia.
19. Discuss research concerning the effects and side effects of antipsychotic medication.
20. Discuss the features of delusional disorder and differentiate the disorder from paranoid schizophrenia and paranoid personality disorder.

KEY TERMS AND CONCEPTS

The following is a list of terms, concepts, and names that are discussed in the chapter. They are important for you to know. Review these terms, comparing your answers with the material presented in the text.

Schizophrenia
Delusions
Hallucinations
Emil Kraeplin
Dementia praecox
Eugen Bleuler
Four A's: association, affect, ambivalence, autism
Schizoaffective disorder
Kurt Schneider
First-rank symptoms
Second-rank symptoms
Prodromal phase
Residual phase
Brief psychotic disorder
Schizophreniform disorder
Schizoaffective disorder
Delusions
Delusions of persecution
Delusions of reference
Delusions of being controlled
Thought broadcasting
Thought insertion
Thought withdrawal
Thought disorder
Neologisms
Perseveration
Clanging
Blocking
Orienting response
Marker
Flat affect
Stupor
Simple schizophrenia
Disorganized type
Catatonic type
Waxy flexibility
Process schizophrenia
Reactive schizophrenia
Prognosis

Negative symptoms
Positive symptoms
Type I
Type II
Primary narcissism
Secondary narcissism
Cross-fostering study
Paul Meehl
Zubin and Spring
Diathesis-stress model
Dopamine theory
Neuroleptics
Phenothiazines
Longitudinal studies
Schizophrenogenic mother
Double-bind communication
Communication deviance
Expressed emotion
Institutionalized syndrome
Tardive dyskinesia
Delusional disorder
Erotomania

MATCHING

Match the following names, terms, and concepts with the definitions listed below. The answers are found at the end of the chapter.

a. schizophreniform disorder
b. markers
c. institutionalization syndrome
d. Emil Kraeplin
e. reactive schizophrenia
f. hallucination
g. hypervigilance
h. second-rank symptoms
i. orienting response
j. perseveration
k. tardive dyskinesia
l. delusion
m. residual phase

n. neuroleptics
o. clanging
p. first-rank symptoms
q. blocking
r. premorbid adjustment
s. schizophrenogenic mother
t. Eugen Bleuler
u. waxy flexibility
v. brief psychotic disorder
w. delusional disorder
x. neologisms
y. prognosis
z. process schizophrenia

1) _____ major tranquilizers that can be helpful in alleviating psychotic symptoms

2) _____ involuntary interruptions of speech

3) _____ introduced the term dementia praecox to describe a medical syndrome characterized by mental and behavioral deterioration

4) _____ a psychotic episode in response to a traumatic event

5) _____ identifiable factors that may predict vulnerability to schizophrenia

6) _____ theorist who characterized schizophrenia as a disorder of the "four A's"

7) _____ word phrases that are strung together that have no meaning but rhyme

8) _____ disorder characterized by delusions without the confused or jumbled thinking and deterioration of behavior of schizophrenia

9) _____ schizophrenic symptoms that have lasted less than six months

10) _____ created words that have no apparent meaning

11) _____ schizophrenia with a clearly identified onset

12) _____ inappropriate and persistent repetition of the same thought

13) _____ the perception of an event in the absence of external stimulation

14) _____ according to Kurt Schneider, symptoms that schizophrenia shared with other disorders

15) _____ level of functioning before the acute phase of schizophrenia

16) _____ acute sensitivity to extraneous stimuli such as sounds

17) _____ the adoption of a fixed posture

18) _____ a cold, aloof, domineering mother who reduces self-esteem and independence

19) _____ return to the previous level of functioning following the acute phase

20) _____ a pattern of passive and dependent behavior in hospitalized persons

21) _____ according to Kurt Schneider, symptoms central to the diagnosis of and unique to schizophrenia

22) _____ the predicted outcome of a disorder

23) _____ a pattern of automatic psychophysiological responses that alerts your brain to the presence of a stimulus

24) _____ a movement disorder created by long term use of antipsychotic drugs

25) _____ a false and illogical belief that cannot be disconfirmed

26) _____ schizophrenia with no clearly identified onset

TRUE-FALSE

The following true-false statements are reprinted here from your text. Can you remember the answers? They can be found at the end of this chapter.

1. _____ Many people with schizophrenia show no emotional response to tragic events.
2. _____ Hallucinations are rare and are almost always a sign of schizophrenia.
3. _____ Auditory hallucinations may be a form of inner speech.
4. _____ Some people with schizophrenia sustain unusual, uncomfortable positions for hours and will not respond to questions or communicate during these periods.
5. _____ A 54-year-old hospitalized woman diagnosed with schizophrenia was conditioned to cling to a broom by being given cigarettes as reinforcers.
6. _____ A child with two parents who have schizophrenia will develop schizophrenia about 90% of the time.
7. _____ People who have schizophrenia were more likely to have been born during the winter than at other times of the year.
8. _____ People with schizophrenia have cold, overprotective mothers.
9. _____ Recent advances in treating schizophrenia have led to a cure in many cases.
10. _____ Some people are deluded that they are loved by a famous person.

MULTIPLE CHOICE

The multiple choice questions listed below will test your understanding of the material presented in the chapter. Read through each question and circle the letter representing the best answer. The answers are found at the end of the chapter.

1) Which of the following features is unique to schizophrenia?

    a. thought disorder
    b. delusions
    c. hallucinations
    d. none of the above features are unique to schizophrenia

2) People who display combined features of schizophrenia and mood disorders are diagnosed with:

    a. brief reactive psychosis
    b. bipolar disorder
    c. schizoaffective disorder
    c. schizophreniform disorder

3) Factors which predict better recovery for schizophrenia include all BUT which of the following?

    a. higher level of premorbid adjustment
    b. earlier age of onset
    c. a more acute onset
    d. intact neurological functioning

4) Which of the following statement is TRUE regarding gender differences in schizophrenia?

    a. men have a less severe course of the disorder
    b. women tend to develop the disorder later
    c. men have achieved a higher level of functioning before the onset of the disorder
    d. all of the above are true

5) Which of the following theorists was heavily influenced by psychodynamic theory?

    a. Kurt Schneider
    b. Eugen Bleuler
    c. Emil Kraeplin
    d. Robert Spitzer

6) Approximately _____ of the world's population will have a schizophrenic episode.

   a. 1-2%
   b. 5-10%
   c. 20%
   d. 25%

7) Negative symptoms of schizophrenia:

   a. reflect a defect in inhibitory mechanisms
   b. are associated with better outcome
   c. appear to reflect the more enduring characteristics of schizophrenia
   d. are less likely to be present between episodes than positive symptoms

8) Which of the following is one of Schneider's first rank symptoms?

   a. disturbances in mood
   b. inappropriate affect
   c. ambivalence
   d. delusions

9) Schizophrenia usually develops at what age?

   a. early childhood
   b. preteen years
   c. late adolescence and early adulthood
   d. middle adulthood

10) Which type of therapy is least effective in the treatment of schizophrenia?

   a. behavioral
   b. biological
   c. psychodynamic
   d. family intervention

11) Which of the following is in the correct order?

   a. acute phase, prodromal phase, residual phase
   b. acute phase, residual phase, prodromal phase
   c. residual phase, prodromal phase, acute phase
   d. prodromal phase, acute phase. residual phase

12) Which of the following statements is true regarding the new drug, clozapine?

    a. it has some adverse side effects which limits its use with schizophrenics
    b. it appears to alleviate only positive symptoms of schizophrenia
    c. it does not affect dopamine receptors in the brain
    d. it does not appear to be an effective medication for schizophrenics

13) A person must show features characteristic of schizophrenia for how long before they are diagnosed as schizophrenic?

    a. 30 days
    b. 3 months
    c. 6 months
    d. 1 year

14) Which of the following features would be LEAST likely to be characteristic of the residual phase of schizophrenia?

    a. deep sense of apathy and indifference
    b. difficulties thinking and speaking clearly
    c. unusual, odd, or eccentric beliefs
    d. flagrant psychotic behaviors

15) The most common type of delusional disorder is the _____ type.

    a. erotomanic
    b. grandiose
    c. jealous
    d. persecutory

16) Which of the following disorders may have a common genetic link with schizophrenia?

    a. schizoid personality disorder
    b. schizoaffective disorder
    c. brief psychotic disorder
    d. borderline personality disorder

17) Which of the following would be an example of a disturbance of volition?

    a. experiencing command hallucinations
    b. lacking interest or drive and unable to pursue a goal
    c. displaying flat affect
    d. speaking in a confused and disordered manner

18) Schizophrenics are:

   a. more likely to be distracted by irrelevant stimuli than nonschizophrenics
   b. less likely to be distracted by irrelevant stimuli than nonschizophrenics
   c. more likely to ignore relevant stimuli than nonschizophrenics
   d. more likely to perseverate on relevant stimuli than nonschizophrenics

19) Believing that one's thoughts are somehow transmitted externally so that other people can hear them is:

   a. delusions of being controlled
   b. delusions of grandeur
   c. thought broadcasting
   d. thought withdrawal

20) Which of the following is NOT one of the types of schizophrenia recognized by the DSM?

   a. simple
   b. disorganized
   c. undifferentiated
   d. paranoid

21) Studies on the genetic component of schizophrenia support that genetic factors account for about _____ of the risk of developing the disorder.

   a. 1/3
   b. 1/2
   c. 3/4
   d. virtually all

22) Ventricular enlargement in schizophrenics is associated with:

   a. greater evidence of negative symptoms
   b. poorer premorbid histories
   c. poorer response to antipsychotic drugs
   d. all of the above

23) The Type I - Type II distinction is similar to the _____ distinction.

   a. reactive-process
   b. simple-undifferentiated
   c. positive-negative symptom
   d. genetic-behavioral

24) Clanging is an example of which type of disturbance?

   a. disturbance in the form of thought
   b. disturbance in the content of thought
   c. disturbance in the level of functioning
   d. deficit in attention

25) If one twin of a pair of monozygotic twins develops schizophrenia, what is the likelihood that the other twin will develop schizophrenia?

   a. less than 10%
   b. 40% - 50%
   c. 70% - 80%
   d. greater than 90%

26) Which of the following would NOT be a component of social skills training for schizophrenics?

   a. psychodrama techniques
   b. role-playing exercises
   c. modeling
   d. direct instruction

27) Birth trauma among _____ children _____ the likelihood that they will develop schizophrenia.

   a. low risk; increases
   b. high risk; increases
   c. low risk; decreases
   d. high risk; decreases

28) Research on brain abnormalities and schizophrenia supports that:

   a. schizophrenics do not have brain abnormalities
   b. many schizophrenics have abnormal occipital lobe activity, resulting in visual hallucinations
   c. many schizophrenics have abnormally low levels of frontal lobe activity
   d. many schizophrenics have neurological deficits caused by viral infections

29) The dopamine theory posits that schizophrenics have dopamine receptors that are:

  a. overreactive
  b. underreactive
  c. blocked
  d. absent

30) A limitation of studying high risk children as a model for the development of schizophrenia is:

  a. high risk children tend to be uncooperative with research
  b. high risk children with a schizophrenic parent have lower IQ scores compared to children without a schizophrenic parent
  c. it is not clear whether the "markers" that characterize high risk children with a schizophrenic parent will generalize to children without a schizophrenic parent
  d. so many high risk children develop schizophrenia that it is difficult to determine valid "markers"

QUESTIONS FOR CRITICAL THINKING

1. Compare the views of Kraeplin, Bleuler, and Schneider. What factors did each emphasize in their definition of schizophrenia?
2. How has the concept of schizophrenia narrowed since the 1950's?
3. How does schizophrenia differ by gender and ethnic group?
4. Discuss the syndrome of Nervios.
5. Discuss the symptoms that are characteristic of schizophrenia. What symptoms are unique to schizophrenia? What symptoms overlap with other disorders?
6. Distinguish process from reactive schizophrenia.
7. Compare positive to negative symptoms. Discuss the research that supports this dimension or subtype.
8. Review the Type I versus Type II dimension of schizophrenia. How valid is this distinction?
9. Discuss the strengths and weaknesses of the psychoanalytic model of schizophrenia.
10. How do longitudinal studies assist in studying schizophrenia?
11. Discuss the research support for the dopamine theory of schizophrenia.
12. Review the literature on brain abnormalities and schizophrenia. What can we say about the possible role of brain abnormalities in the development of schizophrenia.
13. What role do cultural factors play in schizophrenia?
14. Discuss the etiology of tardive dyskinesia. How can it be treated?
15. Discuss the influence of ethnic differences in the treatment of schizophrenia.

16. What are the goals of psychosocial rehabilitation.
17. Distinguish schizophrenia from delusional disorder.
18. How does delusional disorder differ from paranoid personality disorder?

ANSWERS FOR MATCHING

1.	n	10.	x	19.	m
2.	q	11.	e	20.	c
3.	d	12.	j	21.	p
4.	v	13.	f	22.	y
5.	b	14.	h	23.	i
6.	t	15.	r	24.	k
7.	o	16.	g	25.	l
8.	w	17.	u	26.	z
9.	a	18.	s		

TRUE-FALSE ANSWERS

1.	T	6.	F
2.	F	7.	T
3.	T	8.	F
4.	T	9.	F
5.	T	10.	T

MULTIPLE CHOICE ANSWERS

1.	d	11.	d	21.	c
2.	c	12.	a	22.	d
3.	b	13.	c	23.	c
4.	b	14.	d	24.	a
5.	b	15.	d	25.	b
6.	a	16.	b	26.	a
7.	c	17.	b	27.	b
8.	d	18.	a	28.	c
9.	c	19.	c	29.	a
10.	c	20.	a	30.	c

CHAPTER THIRTEEN

ABNORMAL BEHAVIOR IN CHILDHOOD AND ADOLESCENCE

OVERVIEW

This chapter thoroughly outlines the gamet of disorders that can be identified in childhood and adolescence. It begins with a brief discussion of the unique difficulties in diagnosing developmental disorders; that is, the problem of taking into account age, sex, family, and cultural background, and developmental level in assessing the abnormality or normality of a behavior or behaviors. It then continues with a discussion of general risk factors for the disorders of childhood and adolescence. Then, the analysis of the major disorders of childhood and adolescence begins.

There are a number of major disorders discussed in the text. For each disorder, you will need to know four things: the characteristics or definition of the disorder; the risk factors and etiology of the disorders; theories regarding the disorder; and treatment approaches for the disorder.

CHAPTER OUTLINE

Normal and Abnormal in Childhood and Adolescence
Risk Factors for Disorders in Childhood and Adolescence
    Biological Risk Factors
    Psychosocial Risk Factors
Pervasive Developmental Disorders
    Autism
        Theoretical Perspectives
        Treatment
        The Long-term View
Mental Retardation
    Causes of Retardation
        Down Syndrome and Other Chromosomal Abnormalities
        Fragile X Syndrome and Other Genetic Abnormalities
        Prenatal Factors
        Cultural-Familial Causes
        Intervention
Learning Disorders
    Types of Learning Disorders
        Mathematics Disorder
        Disorder of Written Expression
        Reading Disorder
    Theoretical Perspectives
    Intervention

LEARNING OBJECTIVES

The following learning objectives can also be found at the beginning of the chapter. When you have completed your study of the chapter, you should be able to:

1. Discuss ways of determining what is normal and abnormal in childhood and adolescence.
2. Discuss risk factors for disorders in childhood and adolescence.
3. Discuss theoretical perspectives on autism.
4. Differentiate between autism and childhood schizophrenia.
5. Discuss treatment of autism.
6. Describe the assessment of mental retardation.
7. Describe levels of severity of mental retardation.

8. Discuss the causes of mental retardation.
9. Discuss methods of testing for genetic defects.
10. Discuss intervention in cases of mental retardation.
11. Discuss the savant syndrome.
12. Describe types of learning disorders.
13. Discuss theoretical perspectives on learning disorders.
14. Discuss approaches to remediating learning disorders.
15. Describe types of communication disorders.
16. Describe types of disruptive behavior and attention-deficit disorders.
17. Discuss theoretical perspectives on disruptive behavior and attention-deficit disorders.
18. Discuss treatment of disruptive behavior and attention-deficit disorders.
19. Discuss the features and treatment of anxiety disorders affecting children and adolescents.
20. Describe the features and treatment of depression in childhood and adolescence.
21. Discuss the problem of adolescent suicide.
22. Describe the eating disorders of anorexia nervosa and bulimia nervosa.
23. Discuss theoretical perspectives on these eating disorders.
24. Discuss the treatment of these eating disorders.
25. Discuss theoretical perspectives on enuresis and encopresis.
26. Discuss treatment of these disorders.

KEY TERMS AND CONCEPTS

The following is a list of terms, concepts, and names that are discussed in the chapter. They are important for you to know. Review these terms, comparing your answers with the material presented in the text.

Play therapy
Internalized problems
Externalized problems
Psychoses
Autism/Autistic disorder
Eugene Bleuler
Leo Kanner
Bruno Bettelheim
O. Ivar Lovaas
Mental retardation
Down syndrome
Klinefelter's syndrome
Turner's syndrome
Fragile X syndrome
Phenylketonuria

Phenylalanine
Tay-Sachs disease
Amniocentesis
Chorionic villus sampling (CVS)
Cultural-familial mental retardation
Education for All Handicapped Children Act, Public Law 94-142 (PL 94-192)
Developmentally Disabled Assistance and Bill of Rights Act
Time-out
Aversives
Idiot savant/Savant syndrome
Dyslexia
Learning disorder/Learning disability
Mathematics disorder
Disorder of written expression
Reading disorder/Dyslexia
Psychoeducational model
Medical model
Neuropsychological model
Linguistic model
Cognitive model
Communication disorders
Expressive language disorder
Mixed receptive/expressive language disorder
Phonological disorder
Stuttering
Disruptive behavior and attention-deficit disorders
Attention-Deficit/Hyperactivity Disorder (ADHD)
Conduct disorder (CD)
Oppositional defiant disorder (ODD)
Avoidant personality disorder
Separation anxiety disorder
School phobia
Concrete operations
Cuentos
Eating disorders
Anorexia nervosa
Bulimia nervosa
Osteoporosis
Binge-eating disorder
Systems perspective
Enuresis
O. Hobart Mowrer
Bell-and-pad method
Encopresis

MATCHING

Match the following names, terms, and concepts with the definitions listed below. The answers are found at the end of the chapter.

a. cuentos
b. ritalin
c. profound mental retardation
d. dyslexia
e. echolalia
f. aversives
g. Leo Kanner
h. anorexia nervosa
i. Down syndrome
j. enuresis
k. time-out
l. Klinefelter's syndrome
m. O. Ivar Lovaas

n. internalized problems
o. savant syndrome
p. cultural-familial retardation
q. conduct disorder
r. generalized anxiety disorder
s. Fragile X syndrome
t. bulimia nervosa
u. Tay-Sachs disease
v. childhood schizophrenia
w. play therapy
x. encopresis
y. moderate mental retardation
z. externalized problems

1) _____ characterized by confusion, disorientation, incoherent speech, and hallucinations

2) _____ a high-pitched, monotonic repetition of another person's words

3) _____ impoverished social environment producing mental retardation

4) _____ characteristics include a round face, broad flat nose, small hands, and mental retardation

5) _____ includes disorders such as anxiety and depression

6) _____ the most common type of inherited mental retardation

7) _____ a treatment approach in which children enact family conflicts symbolically through their play activities

8) _____ the failure to control one's bowels after the age of 4

9) _____ an IQ score of 35-49 would classify an individual in this category

10) _____ an intense fear of being overweight combined with abnormally low actual weight

11) _____ first to apply the diagnosis of "early infantile autism"

12) _____ a generalized fear or anxiety about past, present, and future events

13) _____ autistic or retarded persons with one exceptional mental ability

14) _____ stories read aloud by therapists or mothers of Puerto Rican children with behavior problems in which the protagonists served as models for adaptive behavior

15) _____ children who purposefully engage in patterns of antisocial behavior that violate social norms and the rights of others may be diagnosed with this

16) _____ an IQ score below 20 would classify an individual in this category

17) _____ a type of punishment, this procedure temporarily removes the child from reinforcing environments

18) _____ characterized by the presence of an extra X sex chromosome, this only occurs in males and results in an XXY sex chromosomal pattern rather than the XY pattern than men normally have

19) _____ the failure to control one's bladder past the age of 5

20) _____ characterizes children who have poorly developed skills in recognizing words and comprehending written text

21) _____ a stimulant drug often used to treat hyperactive children

22) _____ fatal degenerative disease of the central nervous system

23) _____ offered a cognitive-learning perspective on treating autism

24) _____ a recurrent pattern of excessive eating followed by purging

25) _____ includes problems and disorders involving acting out or aggressive behaviors

26) _____ mildly painful stimuli used to control aggressive or destructive behavior

TRUE-FALSE

The following true-false statements are reprinted here from your text. Can you remember the answers? They can be found at the end of this chapter.

1. _____ Many behavior patterns that are normal for children would be considered abnormal among adults.

2. ____ People with severe mental retardation outnumber those with mild retardation by about 2 to 1.
3. ____ Some people can recall verbatim every story they read in a newspaper.
4. ____ Children who are hyperactive are often given stimulants to help calm them down.
5. ____ Some children refuse to go to school because they believe that terrible things may happen to their parents while they are away.
6. ____ Although children and adolescents may sometimes feel sad, it is extremely rare for major depression to arise in childhood and adolescence.
7. ____ Therapists have used Puerto Rican folktales to help Puerto Rican children adjust to the demands of living in mainstream U.S. society.
8. ____ You cannot be too rich or too thin.
9. ____ Even though women with anorexia nervosa may lose a substantial amount of body weight, they continue to menstruate normally.
10. ____ It is normal for children who have acquired daytime control over their bladders to have accidents during the night for a year or more.

MULTIPLE CHOICE

The multiple choice questions listed below will test your understanding of the material presented in the chapter. Read through each question and circle the letter representing the best answer. The answers are found at the end of the chapter.

1) Which of the following disorders affects approximately 3-5% of school-age children and is the most common cause of childhood referrals to mental health agencies?

   a. conduct disorder
   b. depression
   c. anxiety
   d. attention-deficit/hyperactivity disorder

2) Disorders of anxiety and depression in childhood are more likely to be found in _____; in adolescence, they are more likely to be found in _____.

   a. boys; boys
   b. girls; girls
   c. boys; girls
   d. girls; boys

3) In the DSM-IV, childhood schizophrenia:

    a. is diagnosed by markedly different symptoms than adult schizophrenia
    b. is diagnosed by the presence of hallucinations at approximately 20 months of age
    c. was replaced by the name "autistic disorder"
    d. is not a diagnostic classification

4) Research indicates that _____ treatment is effective in improving the IQ scores of autistic children.

    a. behavioral
    b. humanistic-existential
    c. drug
    d. psychodynamic

5) For an individual to be diagnosed as mentally retarded, they must meet three of the following diagnostic criteria. Which of the following is NOT one of the criteria for mental retardation?

    a. IQ of 70 or below
    b. history of aggressive behavior
    c. evidence of the disorder before age 18
    d. impaired adaptive behavior

6) An infant may be placed on a diet low in the protein phenylalanine to prevent mental retardation due to:

    a. Down syndrome
    b. fetal alcohol syndrome
    c. PKU syndrome
    d. cultural-familial retardation

7) Which of the following is true of amniocentesis?

    a. it is a genetic defect causing blindness
    b. it is a blood disease of pregnant women
    c. it a surgical procedure performed 9-12 weeks following conception
    d. it involves drawing fluid from the uterus

8) Treatment based upon which model has produced impressive improvements in the skills of children with learning disabilities?

    a. medical
    b. neuropsychological
    c. psychoeducational
    d. behavioral

9) When a child shows excessive and developmentally inappropriate fear of being removed from his or her mother, the child may be experiencing which disorder?

    a. separation anxiety disorder
    b. conduct disorder
    c. Rhett's disorder
    d. rumination disorder

10) Which of the following is NOT a symptom of childhood depression?

    a. broad negative expectations for the future
    b. underestimating the consequences of negative events
    c. incorrectly assuming responsibility for negative events
    d. selectively attending to negative aspects of events

11) In comparison with normal families, families of anorexics and bulimics show more:

    a. cohesion
    b. emotional expression
    c. conflict
    d. autonomy training

12) Which theoretical perspective suggests that functional enuresis is the result of attempting to toilet train too early?

    a. behavioral
    b. genetic
    c. existential
    d. psychodynamic

13) As an adult, a person can perform simple tasks under sheltered conditions but is incapable of self-maintenance. This person shows _____ mental retardation.

    a. mild
    b. moderate
    c. severe
    d. profound

14) All of the following are examples of externalized problems EXCEPT:

    a. disruptive behavior
    b. depression
    c. aggression
    d. oppositional behavior

15) Which of the following is an example of a communication disorder in DSM-IV?

    a. phonological disorder
    b. reading disorder
    c. expressive writing disorder
    d. none of the above

16) Which of the following disorders is considered a pervasive developmental disorder?

    a. Tourette's syndrome
    b. Autism
    c. selective mutism
    d. expressive language disorder

17) This is characterized by an extra or third chromosome on the 21st pair of chromosomes, resulting in 47 chromosomes rather than the normal complement of 46.

    a. Klinefelter's syndrome
    b. Turner's syndrome
    c. Down syndrome
    d. Tay-Sachs disease

18) All of the following are true of children diagnosed with Attention-Deficit/Hyperactivity Disorder, Combined Type EXCEPT:

    a. they tend to do more poorly in school than their peers
    b. they tend to fidget or squirm in their seats
    c. they tend to be popular with classmates because they are so outgoing
    d. they tend to have difficulty following through on instructions

19) Which of the following factors is NOT associated with an increased risk of suicide among children and adolescents?

    a. gender
    b. age
    c. race
    d. all of the above are risk factors

20) The average age of onset for bulimia is:

    a. pre-teenage years
    b. early teenage years
    c. late teenage years
    d. late-twenties to early-thirties

21) In Mowrer's bell-and-pad method for treating nocturnal enuresis in children, the technique is usually explained through principles of:

    a. operant conditioning
    b. classical conditioning
    c. behavioral modification
    d. aversive training

22) The special skills demonstrated by savants are usually associated with which brain functions?

    a. right hemisphere
    b. left hemisphere
    c. hypothalamic
    d. occipital cortex

23) Which of the following is NOT a feature of major depression among children and adolescents?

    a. sense of hopelessness
    b. lower self-esteem
    c. increased appetite
    d. fatigue

24) All of the following are diagnostic features of autism EXCEPT:

    a. impaired communication
    b. impaired inhibitory system
    c. impaired social interactions
    d. restricted, repetitive and stereotyped behavior patterns

25) Which of the following is NOT a medical complication of anorexia?

    a. neurological problems
    b. dermatological problems
    c. cardiovascular complications
    d. gastrointestinal problems

26) Symptoms of Attention-Deficit/Hyperactivity Disorder have been linked to:

   a. sugar intake
   b. poor nutrition
   c. artificial sweeteners
   d. none of the above

27) _____ is (are) common among adolescents, but _____ is (are) not.

   a. generalized anxiety disorder; obsessive-compulsive disorder
   b. obsessive-compulsive disorder; generalized anxiety disorder
   c. depressive disorders; anxiety disorders
   d. anxiety disorders; depressive disorders

28) The average length of a major depressive episode in childhood or adolescence is approximately:

   a. 1 month
   b. 6 months
   c. 11 months
   d. 24 months

29) Autism is caused by:

   a. poor parenting
   b. an economically deprived background
   c. poor prenatal care
   d. the causes remain unknown

30) Current research indicates that _____ seems to be the most effective treatment for Attention-Deficit/Hyperactivity Disorder.

   a. play therapy
   b. social skills training
   c. stimulant medication
   d. all of the above

QUESTIONS FOR CRITICAL THINKING

1. Describe how normal behavior in childhood and adolescence differ from abnormal behavior.
2. Discuss the history of and current thinking about the etiology of autistic disorder.
3. Discuss how genetic counseling is used.

4. Discuss why mainstreaming is controversial. What is your personal opinion about this? Where do you think your beliefs on this topic originated?

5. Describe the types of attention-deficit and disruptive behavior disorders and the types of treatment most effective for working with children and adolescents diagnosed with these disorders.

6. Discuss the features and treatment of anxiety disorders affecting children and adolescents.

7. Describe the features and treatment of depression in children and adolescents.

8. Identify the risk factors and discuss the research on adolescent suicide.

9. Compare and contrast anorexia nervosa with bulimia nervosa.

10. Discuss the role that the family plays in eating disorders.

11. Discuss how the cultural ideal has affected attitudes about body image.

12. Using Mowrer's bell-and-pad method, describe how you would treat a 10-year-old male presenting with a diagnosis of nocturnal enuresis.

ANSWERS FOR MATCHING

1.	v	10.	h	19.	j		
2.	e	11.	g	20.	d		
3.	p	12.	r	21.	b		
4.	i	13.	o	22.	u		
5.	n	14.	a	23.	m		
6.	s	15.	q	24.	t		
7.	w	16.	c	25.	z		
8.	x	17.	k	26.	f		
9.	y	18.	l				

TRUE-FALSE ANSWERS

1.	T	4.	T	7.	T
2.	F	5.	T	8.	F
3.	T	6.	F	9.	F
				10.	T

MULTIPLE CHOICE ANSWERS

1.	d	11.	c	21.	b
2.	c	12.	a	22.	a
3.	d	13.	b	23.	c
4.	a	14.	b	24.	b
5.	b	15.	a	25.	a
6.	c	16.	b	26.	d
7.	d	17.	c	27.	a
8.	d	18.	c	28.	c
9.	a	19.	d	29.	d
10.	b	20.	c	30.	c

CHAPTER FOURTEEN

COGNITIVE DISORDERS AND DISORDERS RELATED TO AGING

OVERVIEW

This chapter addresses some of the many ways in which thinking, memory, judgement, and mood disturbances are affected by physical problems. Major types of cognitive disorders include delirium, dementia, and amnestic disorders. Delirium and dementia can be induced by a variety of injuries, infections, and diseases. Amnestic disorders involve organically induced memory deficits; one major type can be produced by prolonged heavy consumption of alcohol. After the chapter reviews delirium, dementia, amnestic disorders, and their major causes, it closes with consideration of epilepsy, a condition that has been much misunderstood throughout history. Types and treatment of epilepsy are described.

CHAPTER OUTLINE

Cognitive Disorders
Classification of Cognitive Disorders
Diagnostic Problems
Delirium
The DTs
Amnestic Disorders
Alcohol-Induced Persisting Amnestic Disorder (Korsakoff's Syndrome)
Dementia
Psychological Disorders Related to Aging
Cognitive Changes in Later Life
Anxiety Disorders and Aging
Depression and Aging
Memory Functioning and Depression
Treating Depression in Older People
Sleep Problems and Aging
Dementia of the Alzheimer's Type
Diagnosis
Features of Alzheimer's Disease
Impact on the Family: A Funeral That Never Ends
Theoretical Perspectives
Treatment
Vascular Dementia
Features of Vascular Dementia
Strokes and Vascular Dementia
Dementias and Other Psychological Problems Due to General Medical Conditions
Dementia Due to Pick's Disease

LEARNING OBJECTIVES

The following learning objectives can also be found at the beginning of the chapter. When you have completed your study of the chapter, you should be able to:

1. Discuss the basic features of cognitive disorders and how they are classified.
2. Discuss problems in diagnosing cognitive disorders.
3. Define delirium and discuss the causes of various kinds of delirium, including the DTs.
4. Discuss the features and causes of amnestic disorders.
5. Discuss the origins and features of Korsakoff's syndrome.
6. Discuss the basic features of dementia and the relationship between dementia and aging.
7. Discuss the cognitive changes associated with aging.
8. Discuss problems relating to anxiety and depression among older people, including relationships between memory problems and depression.
9. Discuss the incidence and features of Alzheimer's disease.
10. Discuss the impact of Alzheimer's disease on the family.
11. Discuss theoretical perspectives on Alzheimer's disease on the family.
12. Discuss the features of vascular dementia.
13. Discuss the features of dementia due to Pick's disease.
14. Discuss the features, origins, and treatment of Parkinson's disease.
15. Discuss the features and origins of Huntington's disease.

16. Discuss the dementias due to HIV disease and Creutzfeldt-Jakob disease.
17. Discuss the dementia and other psychological problems resulting from the different types of head trauma.
18. Discuss the psychological effects associated with brain tumors.
19. Discuss the psychological features associated with nutritional disorders.
20. Discuss the psychological effects of endocrine disorders.
21. Discuss the psychological effects resulting from infections of the brain.

KEY TERMS AND CONCEPTS

The following is a list of terms, concepts, and names that are discussed in the chapter. They are important for you to know. Review these terms, comparing your answers with the material presented in the text.

Oliver Sacks
Tactile information
Agnosia
Delirium
Amnestic disorders
Delirium tremens
Hypoxia
Infarction
Alcohol-induced persisting amnestic disorder (Korsakoff's syndrome)
Wernicke's disease
Ataxia
Dementia
Aphasia
Apraxia
Agnosia
Senile dementia
Presenile dementia
Sleep apnea
Alzheimer's disease
Alois Alzheimer
Beta-amyloid
Cerebrovascular accident
Multi-infarct dementia
Cerebral thrombrosis
Cerebral embolism
Atherosclerosis
Cerebral hemorrhage
Pick's disease
Parkinson's disease
Sustantia nigra

L-dopa
Huntington's disease
GABA
Choreiform movements
Human immunodeficiency virus
Creutzfeldt-Jacob disease
Concussion
Contusion
Laceration
Cerebral hemorrhage
Pellagra
Beriberi
Thyroxin
Hyperthyroidism (Grave's disease)
Cretinism
Hypothyroidism
Addison's disease
Cushing's syndrome
Encephalitis
Meningitis
General paresis
Epilepsy
Acquired or symptomatic epilepsy
Idiopathic epilepsy
Tonic-clonic epilepsy
Grand mal seizure
Tonic phase
Clonic phase
Petit mal epilepsy
Petit mal seizure
Psychomotor or temporal lobe epilepsy

MATCHING

Match the following names, terms, and concepts with the definitions listed below. The answers are found at the end of the chapter.

a. delirium tremens
b. petit mal epilepsy
c. Addison's disease
d. encephalitis
e. Parkinson's disease
f. cretinism
g. laceration
h. acquired epilepsy
i. cerebral hemorrhage
j. agnosia
k. dementia
l. meningitis
m. grand mal seizure

n. Cushing's syndrome
o. aphasia
p. cerebrovascular disorder
q. stroke
r. alcohol persisting amnestic disorder
s. concussion
t. multi-infarct dementia
u. thyroxin
v. tonic-clonic epilepsy
w. contusion
x. general paresis
y. basal ganglia
z. pellagra

1) _____ brain damage due to the blockage of a blood vessel

2) _____ characterized by shaking, tremors, abnormal posture and lack of control over movements

3) _____ brain injury caused by a foreign object piercing the skull

4) _____ inflammation of the membranes that cover the spinal cord and brain

5) _____ a form of physical and mental deterioration that results from neurosyphilis

6) _____ brain trauma caused by a hard blow producing loss of consciousness

7) _____ brain disorder caused by vascular accident

8) _____ inability to recognize objects despite an intact sensory system

9) _____ loss of ability to speak or understand speech

10) _____ dementia caused by small repeated strokes

11) _____ vitamin B deficiency producing anxiety, depression, and memory loss

12) _____ group of cell bodies which lie under the cortex and control motor behavior

13) _____ delirium caused by abrupt withdrawal from alcohol

14) _____ substance secreted by thyroid gland

15) _____ results in loss of consciousness, convulsive and jerking movements, and memory loss

16) _____ bruising of the brain caused by a hard blow

17) _____ epilepsy characterized by grand mal seizures

18) _____ disorder caused by decreased activity in the adrenal cortex, characterized by weight loss, low blood pressure, fatigue, irritability, and depression

19) _____ inflammation of the brain

20) _____ damage produced by blood vessels rupturing, causing blood to leak into the brain

21) _____ disorder caused by overactivity of the adrenal cortex, characterized by weight gain, fatigue, muscle weakness, and negative mood

22) _____ short and long term memory loss due to chronic alcohol abuse

23) _____ epilepsy due to known causes

24) _____ stunted growth and mental retardation produced by hypothryroidism

25) _____ an abnormal and significant decline in intellectual functioning

26) _____ characterized by involuntary lapses in consciousness without motor involvement

TRUE-FALSE

The following true-false statements are reprinted here from your text. Can you remember the answers? They can be found at the end of this chapter.

1. _____ A man with a brain tumor patted the heads of fire hydrants and parking meters in the belief that they were children.
2. _____ The most frequently identified cause of delirium is abrupt withdrawal from alcohol or other drugs.
3. _____ After a motorcycle accident, a medical student failed to recognize the woman he had married a few weeks earlier.

4. ____ Dementia is a normal function of the aging process.
5. ____ Depression often goes undiagnosed in older adults.
6. ____ Alzheimer's disease is found only among older people.
7. ____ Alzheimer's disease is caused by aluminum ingestion.
8. ____ Football players and prize-fighters can recover completely-- display no lingering cognitive deficits from being knocked out.
9. ____ When the symptoms of syphilis disappear by themselves, there is nothing to be concerned about.
10. ____ Julius Caesar and Vincent van Gogh suffered from epilepsy.

MULTIPLE CHOICE

The multiple choice questions listed below will test your understanding of the material presented in the chapter. Read through each question and circle the letter representing the best answer. The answers are found at the end of the chapter.

1) The diagnosis of Alzheimer's disease depends upon finding which of the following?

    a. abnormal loss of memory
    b. inability to manage everyday tasks
    c. neurotic plaques and neurofibrillary tangles
    d. basal ganglia atrophy

2) Diagnosis of cognitive disorders can be difficult because:

    a. damage to the same area of the brain may result in different symptoms for different people
    b. abnormal behavior patterns found in cognitive disorders resemble those occurring in other mental disorders such as depression
    c. brain damage may result in a variety of symptoms
    d. all of the above

3) Which disorder is a progressive dementia that is similar to Alzheimer's disease and is additionally characterized by social inappropriateness such as the display of flagrant sexual behavior?

    a. Parkinson's disease
    b. Cushing's syndrome
    c. Pick's disease
    d. Huntington's disease

4) Parkinson's disease involves the destruction of brain cells in which area of the brain?

        a. substantia nigra
        b. basal ganglia
        c. cerebral cortex
        d. temporal lobe

5) Which of the following is NOT a symptom of delirium?

        a. disorientation to time and place
        b. apprehension, fear, or panic
        c. delusions or hallucinations
        d. persistent, irreversible decline in memory

6) Which type of knowledge or memory appears to be fairly resistant to the aging process?

        a. memory associated with timed performance tasks
        b. interpersonal memory
        c. vocabulary and accumulated knowledge
        d. fluid memory

7) Which of the following is NOT one of the three major types of cognitive disorders?

        a. alcohol-induced disorders
        b. delirium
        c. dementia
        d. amnestic disorders

8) The son or daughter of an Alzheimer's victim is _____ likely to get Alzheimer's as a person whose parent does or did not have Alzheimer's.

        a. less
        b. no more
        c. four times more
        d. ten times more

9) Which pair of the following medications is typically used to control the occurrence of seizures in epileptics?

        a. Dilantin and Ritalin
        b. Dilantin and phenobarbital
        c. phenobarbital and benzodiazapene
        d. L-dopa and phenobarbital

10) Which of the following statements is FALSE according to the Attitudes Toward Aging Questionnaire?

    a. the occupational performance of the older worker is typically less effective than that of the younger adult
    b. by age 60 most couples have lost their capacity for satisfying sexual relations
    c. most older people are depressed much of the time
    d. all of the above are false

11) Which of the following is a possible cause of delirium?

    a. abnormally low levels of thyroxin at birth
    b. an abnormal chromosome
    c. fluid or electrolyte imbalances
    d. the presence of neurofibrillary tangles

12) Which of the following statements regarding HIV infection and dementia is true?
    a. HIV infected persons with some form of dementia tend to decline faster and die sooner compared to those persons without dementia
    b. cognitive impairment typically manifests itself before the AIDS stage of HIV infection
    c. HIV infected persons without dementia tend to decline faster and die sooner compared to those persons without dementia
    d. The first signs of dementia due to HIV disease may mimic the DTs

13) Approximately _____% of the population over age 85 suffer from dementia.

    a. 10
    b. 20
    c. 40
    d. 50

14) Which of the following statements about epilepsy is true?

    a. having a seizure is a sure diagnostic sign that one has epilepsy
    b. epilepsy produces profound personality disturbances
    c. idiopathic epilepsy is a genetic disorder
    d. most epileptics do NOT require custodial care

15) Which statement is TRUE regarding cognitive disorders?

    a. they involve disturbances in thinking or memory that represent a significant change from the person's prior functioning
    b. they are caused by medical conditions or drug use or withdrawal that affect brain functioning
    c. they can be short-lived and reversible or chronic and enduring
    d. all of the above

16) Which of the following is NOT a risk factor for depression in older people?

    a. poor health
    b. living alone
    c. lower intelligence level
    d. lower income level

17) Huntington's disease produces all BUT which of the following symptoms?

    a. jerky movements
    b. unstable mood
    c. violent behavior
    d. memory loss

18) Amnestic disorders are characterized by:

    a. the presence of seizures
    b. profound personality change
    c. deficits in either short or long-term memory
    d. gradual decline in intelligence

19) Persons with _____ epilepsy retain control of their motor functions but lose contact with reality.

    a. tonic-clonic
    b. symptomatic
    c. focal
    d. temporal lobe

20) Which of the following is NOT a feature of Alzheimer's disease?

    a. wandering
    b. agitation and aggression
    c. choreiform movements
    d. suspicion, paranoia, and psychotic behavior

21) Approximately _____ % of the children of a person who has Huntington's disease will also contract the disease.

   a. 100
   b. 50
   c. 10
   d. 1

22) Which of the following is another name for alcohol amnestic syndrome?

   a. Wernicke's disease
   b. beriberi
   c. Korsakoff's syndrome
   d. Pick's disease

23) Research on depression in the elderly supports which of the following?

   a. caregivers of elderly people suffering from dementia are at risk for depression
   b. depression in the elderly is easily recognized by physicians
   c. people who retire voluntarily are not at risk for depression
   d. all of the above

24) An amnestic disorder frequently appears following:

   a. a psychologically traumatic event
   b. a blow to the head
   c. a serious physical illness
   d. ingestion of a drug

25) Research on the treatment of depression in the elderly suggests that:

   a. psychotherapy can be a very effective form of treatment
   b. drugs are the best treatment for elderly depressed people
   c. psychotherapy is not appropriate for elderly people
   d. electro-convulsive shock treatment (ECT) is the most effective form of treatment for depressed elderly people

26) Brain tumors can produce which of the following symptoms?

   a. loss of memory and disorientation
   b. impaired motor coordination and seizures
   c. personality changes and hallucinations
   d. all of the above can be produced by brain tumors

27) Which of the following statements is NOT true regarding dementia?

    a. it is typically progressive and irreversible
    b. the cognitive decline is typically less rapid and severe compared to normal aging
    c. it most often affects people in later life
    d. there are more than 70 known causes

28) How are cognitive disorders classified in DSM-IV?

    a. the disorder is classified on Axis I, the medical condition is classified on Axis II
    b. the disorder is classified on Axis I, the medical condition is classified on Axis III
    c. the disorder is classified on Axis I, the medical condition is classified on Axis IV
    d. the disorder is classified on Axis II, the medical condition is classified on Axis IV

29) Chronic alcoholism may be a contributing factor in:

    a. Grave's disease
    b. beriberi
    c. Addison's disease
    d. all of the above

30) When asked, Joe can tell his doctor how to button a shirt, but cannot button his own shirt when asked to do so. Joe may have which of the following deficits?

    a. aphasia
    b. hypoxia
    c. apraxia
    d. agnosia

QUESTIONS FOR CRITICAL THINKING

1.   What are the diagnostic problems with cognitive disorders?
2.   How do delirium and dementia differ?
3.   How does normal aging differ from mild and moderate Alzheimer's Disease?
4.   Why do some people describe Alzheimer's Disease as "a funeral that never ends"?
5.   How does multi-infarct dementia differ from Alzheimer's Disease?
6.   How is dementia related to HIV infection and AIDS?

7. Describe the similarities and differences between Pick's Disease, Parkinson's Disease, and Huntington's Disease. What are the ways in which these conditions are treated?
8. What can cause an amnestic disorder?
9. What types of sleep disorders are common in elderly people?
10. Is epilepsy a disease in itself? Describe the characteristic features of the different types.
11. Distinguish the myths from the facts about epilepsy.

ANSWERS FOR MATCHING

1.	q	10.	t	19.	d
2.	e	11.	z	20.	i
3.	g	12.	y	21.	n
4.	l	13.	a	22.	r
5.	x	14.	u	23.	h
6.	s	15.	m	24.	f
7.	p	16.	w	25.	k
8.	j	17.	v	26.	b
9.	o	18.	c		

TRUE-FALSE ANSWERS

1.	T	6.	F
2.	T	7.	F
3.	T	8.	T
4.	F	9.	F
5.	T	10.	T

MULTIPLE CHOICE ANSWERS

1.	c	11.	c	21.	b
2.	d	12.	a	22.	c
3.	c	13.	b	23.	a
4.	a	14.	d	24.	b
5.	d	15.	d	25.	a
6.	c	16.	c	26.	d
7.	a	17.	c	27.	b
8.	c	18.	c	28.	b
9.	b	19.	d	29.	b
10.	d	20.	c	30.	c

CHAPTER FIFTEEN

VIOLENCE AND ABUSE

OVERVIEW

This chapter focuses on violence and abusive behaviors, problems that are perhaps more serious in our country than in most other civilized countries of the world. The chapter reviews different theories of aggression, then discusses specific factors such as alcohol that may contribute to aggressive behavior in our society.

The chapter continues by outlining different forms of violence that are serious problems, including spouse abuse, child abuse, rape, and child sexual abuse. It is important to note that the persons who commit such aggressive acts do not receive a particular DSM diagnosis. That is, they are not necessarily considered mentally ill. However, the acts they commit can have serious psychological consequences for the victim. Treatment strategies for both offenders and victims are discussed. The chapter ends by defining and reviewing types of sexual harassment.

CHAPTER OUTLINE

Violence and Abnormal Behavior
       Violence and Psychological Disorders
Perspectives on Aggression
       Biological Perspectives
              Sociobiological Views
              Neurobiological Bases of Aggression
       Social-Learning Perspectives
       Cognitive Perspectives
       Sociocultural Perspectives
              Homicide Rates and Ethnicity
       Alcohol and Aggression
       Emotional Factors in Violent Behavior
       Multiple Causation in Human Aggression
Spouse Abuse
       Psychological Characteristics of Male Batterers
       Patterns of Abuse
       Sociocultural Viewpoints
       Effects of Spouse Abuse
       Why Don't Battered Women Just Leave?
       Treatment of Batterers and Abused Spouses
Child Abuse
       What is Child Abuse?
       Factors in Child Abuse

LEARNING OBJECTIVES

The following learning objectives can also be found at the beginning of the chapter. When you have completed your study of the chapter, you should be able to:

1. Discuss the conditions under which violent behavior may be classified as either normal or abnormal.
2. Discuss the relationship between violent behavior and psychological disorders.
3. Discuss biological, social-learning, cognitive, and sociocultural perspectives on aggression.
4. Discuss the relationship between alcohol use and aggression.
5. Discuss relationships between anger, frustration, and aggression.
6. Discuss the multiple causes that are believed to play a role in human aggression and how they may interact.
7. Discuss the incidence of spouse abuse in the United States and in relation to ethnicity and socioeconomic level.
8. Discuss the psychological characteristics of spouse abusers.
9. Describe the patterns of spouse abuse.

10. Describe sociocultural viewpoints on spouse abuse.
11. Discuss the effects of spouse abuse.
12. Discuss how trauma may impair a battered woman's ability to cope.
13. Discuss approaches to treating batterers and abused spouses.
14. Discuss the different types of child abuse and the prevalence of child abuse in the United States.
15. Describe factors that increase the risk of child abuse.
16. Discuss an integrative approach to understanding child maltreatment.
17. Discuss the effects of child abuse, as well as child abuse treatment and prevention efforts.
18. Discuss the incidence of rape and theoretical perspectives on its causes.
19. Discuss the effects of rape on survivors.
20. Discuss the treatment of rape survivors and of rapists.
21. Describe the prevalence and patterns of child sexual abuse, and the characteristics of abusers.
22. Discuss the effects of child sexual abuse, treatment of survivors, and efforts at prevention.
23. Discuss approaches to treating rapists and child molesters.
24. Discuss the types, prevalence, and effects of sexual harassment.

KEY TERMS AND CONCEPTS

The following is a list of terms, concepts, and names that are discussed in the chapter. They are important for you to know. Review these terms, comparing your answers with the material presented in the text.

Instinct
Catharsis
Sociobiology
Frustration
Frustration-aggression hypothesis
Battered-woman syndrome
Sexual aggression
Forcible rape
Statutory rape
Stranger rape
Date rape
Empathy training
Sexual harassment

MATCHING

Match the following names, terms, and concepts with the definitions listed below. The answers are found at the end of the chapter.

a. stranger rape
b. sociobiology
c. thought conversion
d. antiandrogen drugs
e. sexual harassment
f. anger management training
g. cognitive theory of aggression
h. date rape
i. instinct
j. physical abuse
k. empathy training
l. sexual aggression
m. death instinct

n. catharsis
o. statutory rape
p. emotional maltreatment
q. battered woman syndrome
r. hypothalamus
s. biological theory of aggression
t. serotonin
u. frustration
v. disinhibition
w. social-learning theory of aggression
x. physical neglect
y. forcible rape
z. frustration-aggression hypothesis

1) _____ the emotion associated with the thwarting of one's attempts to achieve a goal

2) _____ according to Freud, an underlying instinct for human aggression

3) _____ a term describing both acts of outright sexual violence as well as sexual harassment

4) _____ an area of the brain that may regulate aggressive behavior

5) _____ training that attempts to increase an offender's sensitivity toward his victim

6) _____ a term used to describe the traumatizing effects of battering

7) _____ constant harsh criticism of a child involving verbally abusive language or emotional neglect

8) _____ a form of sexual coercion in which a person subjects another person to unwanted sexual comments, gestures, physical contact, overtures, or direct demands for sexual favors

9) _____ a theory emphasizing the role of emotional factors in aggressive behavior

10) _____ the process that involves the loosening of inhibitions or restraints that normally constrain impulsive behavior

11) _____ a cognitive-behavioral treatment approach that helps people identify and correct anger-inducing thoughts and experiences in various situations

12) _____ proposes that aggressive behavior is learned through modeling and reinforcement

13) _____ failure to provide a child with, or withholding from them basic resources such as food, shelter, and medical care needed to promote growth and development

14) _____ a term used to describe the act of rape performed by someone whom the victim has not met or does not know

15) _____ biological treatment for sex offenders that reduces testosterone production

16) _____ an inborn pattern of behavior

17) _____ the use of force, violence, or threats to coerce someone into sexual intercourse

18) _____ the venting of intense emotions or impulses

19) _____ a theory that emphasizes how people interpret confrontative and conflict situations in explaining aggression

20) _____ an inhibitory neurotransmitter that curbs central nervous system activity

21) _____ nonaccidental physical injury of a child, ranging from superficial bruises to death resulting from severe physical injuries

22) _____ the theory that aggressive behavior is an inborn pattern of behavior serving a survival function

23) _____ a specific form of acquaintance rape

24) _____ the doctrine that proposes that behavioral traits, like physical traits, can be transmitted genetically

25) _____ the process of attitude change that allows captors or victims to view their tormentors in sympathetic terms

26) _____ sexual intercourse with someone who is unable to give consent, such as a child or someone with a mental disability

TRUE-FALSE

The following true-false statements are reprinted here from your text. Can you remember the answers? They can be found at the end of this chapter.

1. _____ Alcohol is involved in half the homicides committed in the United States.
2. _____ Spouse abuse contributes to the problem of homelessness in our society.
3. _____ Women who remain with men who abuse them are masochistic.
4. _____ People who were abused as children are likely to abuse their own children.
5. _____ On the average, a rape occurs every 5 minutes in the United States.
6. _____ The majority of rapes are committed by strangers in deserted neighborhoods or darkened alleyways.
7. _____ Some people are sexually aroused by violence.
8. _____ Most rapists are mentally ill.
9. _____ Physical force is seldom used in sexual assaults of children.
10. _____ In some cases, sexual relations between clients and therapists are therapeutically justified.

MULTIPLE CHOICE

The multiple choice questions listed below will test your understanding of the material presented in the chapter. Read through each question and circle the letter representing the best answer. The answers are found at the end of the chapter.

1) Which of the following statements is TRUE regarding childhood sexual abuse?

   a. family members who discover that a child has been abused by a family member are much more likely to report the abuse
   b. the great majority of cases of sexual abuse involve someone who has some kind of relationship with the child
   c. gay males and lesbians account for a disproportionate number of child sexual abusers
   d. most fathers who sexually abuse daughters have a satisfying marital relationship

2) Violent behavior is considered abnormal if:

   a. it occurs outside a socially sanctioned context and if it is harmful to one's self or others
   b. it occurs within a socially sanctioned context but ends up being harmful to one's self or others
   c. it occurs repeatedly across different situations
   d. it occurs without the consent of the person the behavior is directed toward

3) An example of a rational alternative statement to the angering self-statement "No one should be allowed to treat me this way. I'm going to make him sorry real fast" is:

    a. "Relax. People are not always going to be considerate. I don't need to take it personally."
    b. "Relax. I know the boss and I can get him fired anyway."
    c. "I better wait until he leaves work. If I'm still mad I'll jump him on the street."
    d. "He's such a nerd it's not worth getting upset over."

4) The most common form of child abuse is:

    a. physical abuse
    b. sexual abuse
    c. emotional maltreatment
    d. neglect

5) Which of the following is NOT considered a factor that may affect a battered woman's ability to cope effectively?

    a. stress-related reactions
    b. lack of financial resources
    c. difficulties handling troubling emotions
    d. learned helplessness

6) An important contributing factor to the high rate of homicides in our country is:

    a. the ethnic diversity represented in our country
    b. the disproportionate number of poor in our country
    c. easy access to firearms
    d. all of the above

7) Research on the effects of media violence suggests which of the following?

    a. TV violence does not contribute to aggressive behavior
    b. TV violence contributes to aggressive behavior but aggressive children are also more likely to watch it; that is, a circular relationship exists
    c. aggressive children are less likely to watch TV violence because they are quickly bored by it
    d. a supportive family does not mitigate the effect of TV violence

8) Which of the following would NOT be considered a rape prevention strategy for women?

    a. keeping the car doors locked and windows rolled up
    b. having keys handy for the car or front door
    c. walking alone after dark
    d. using one's full name in the phone directory

9) Approximately what percent of people with psychological disorders are also violent?

    a. 10%
    b. 25%
    c. 50%
    d. 90%

10) That domestic violence is a product of the differential power relationships that exist between men and women in our society is a viewpoint of which theoretical perspective?

    a. cognitive perspective
    b. biological perspective
    c. learning theory perspective
    d. sociocultural perspective

11) Which of the following is a risk factor for childhood sexual abuse?

    a. ethnic background
    b. social class
    c. less cohesive family
    d. children under the age of five

12) Which psychological disorder is associated with a higher risk for violent behavior?

    a. depression
    b. antisocial personality disorder
    c. schizophrenia
    d. narcissistic personality disorder

13) An important risk factor for child abuse is:

    a. parental stress
    b. personality of the child
    c. lack of previous abuse in the home
    d. all of the above

14) Sociocultural research on violence suggests that all BUT which of the following may contribute to violent behavior?

    a. cultural acceptance of aggressive behavior
    b. gang subculture
    c. higher levels of testosterone in men
    d. social stressors such as unemployment in the home

15) The most widely used form of treatment for sex offenders who are in prison is:
    a. most offenders receive little or nothing in the way of psychological treatment in prison
    b. biologically based treatments such as castration
    c. individual psychotherapy
    d. social skills training

16) Which of the following statements is TRUE regarding rape survivors?

    a. rape survivors only benefit from short-term treatment immediately following the rape itself
    b. most rape survivors receive prompt attention from mental health professionals, crisis teams, and other resources following the rape
    c. rape survivors with adequate social support do not need additional treatment
    d. most rape survivors do not seek help from mental health professionals, crisis centers or other resources

17) Which of the following is NOT one of the factors to consider in understanding the development of child abuse as outlined by Jay Belsky?

    a. developmental context
    b. immediate interactional context
    c. physical context
    d. community or cultural context

18) Which of the following statements about spouse abuse is TRUE?

   a. men are much more likely to sustain physical injuries
   b. men are much more likely to physically abuse their spouses
   c. women are much more likely to receive physical abuse from their spouses
   d. women are about as likely to physically abuse their husbands as the reverse

19) Which is NOT an example of sexual harassment?

   a. brushing against a person's body
   b. remarks about a person's body or clothing
   c. forced sexual intercourse
   d. verbal harassment

20) More than half of the rapes committed in this country are against which of the following groups?

   a. females under the age of 18
   b. females between the ages of 18 and 30
   c. females between the ages of 30 and 50
   d. females over the age of 50

21) About one-half of the murder victims in the United States are:

   a. non-Hispanic White Americans
   b. African Americans
   c. Asian Americans
   d. Hispanic Americans

22) Characteristics associated with male batterers include which of the following?

   a. higher income level
   b. lower levels of stress
   c. lack of assertive self-expression
   d. higher educational status

23) PTSD, depression, physical health problems, and sexual dysfunction are possible consequences of which of the following?

   a. emotional neglect
   b. rape
   c. chronic marital relationship dysfunction
   d. sexual harassment

24) Which of the following characterizes persons who were abused during childhood?

 a. more likely to engage in criminal violence
 b. more likely to have been arrested during adolescence and adulthood
 c. more likely to be less educated and to hold lower paying jobs
 d. all of the above

25) Alcohol may contribute to aggressive behavior in which of the following ways?

 a. it has a relaxing effect that may make a person less sensitive to cues that serve to inhibit aggressive behavior
 b. it reduces the capacity to weigh the consequences of one's behavior, which may lead to aggressive behavior
 c. it increases the likelihood of misreading the motives of others, which may then lead to aggression
 d. all of the above

QUESTIONS FOR CRITICAL THINKING

1. Describe the relationship between violent behavior and psychological disorder.
2. Compare the following theories of aggression: biological, social-learning, cognitive, and sociocultural. Which theory do you find most comprehensive in its explanation of aggression? Why?
3. Discuss the effects of TV violence on children.
4. Discuss the relationship between alcohol use and violence.
5. Who is most likely to suffer from spouse abuse?
6. Describe the psychological profile of a male batterer.
7. Review the psychological factors that may affect a battered woman's ability to cope effectively.
8. Discuss the parental factors that are associated with increased risk for child abuse.
9. What are the common psychological and physical effects of child abuse?
10. What progress has been made in treating the parents and the children involved in child abuse?
11. Describe the risk factors for rape.
12. Discuss the cultural myths that support rape in our society.
13. Review the two-phase treatment for rape survivors.
14. What are the steps that can be taken to prevent child abuse?
15. Describe the treatment approaches that have been used for sex offenders?
16. Why do you think sexual harassment is so prevalent in our society?
17. What are the effects of sexual harassment?

ANSWERS FOR MATCHING

1.	u	10.	v	19.	g
2.	m	11.	f	20.	t
3.	l	12.	w	21.	j
4.	r	13.	x	22.	s
5.	k	14.	a	23.	h
6.	q	15.	d	24.	b
7.	p	16.	i	25.	c
8.	e	17.	y	26.	o
9.	z	18.	n		

TRUE-FALSE ANSWERS

1.	T	6.	F
2.	T	7.	T
3.	F	8.	F
4.	F	9.	T
5.	F	10.	F

MULTIPLE CHOICE ANSWERS

1.	b	11.	c	21.	b
2.	a	12.	b	22.	c
3.	a	13.	a	23.	b
4.	d	14.	c	24.	d
5.	b	15.	a	25.	d
6.	c	16.	d		
7.	b	17.	c		
8.	d	18.	d		
9.	a	19.	c		
10.	d	20.	a		

CHAPTER SIXTEEN

ABNORMAL PSYCHOLOGY AND SOCIETY:
LEGAL ISSUES AND THE CHALLENGE OF PREVENTION

OVERVIEW

The major issues of this chapter involve legal issues. The first six sections cover legal obligations and conflicts for persons in helping professions. The last section covers two challenges facing helping professionals.

The first two sections examine two tasks that confront helping professionals. The first, "Psychiatric Commitment", discusses the conditions under which people can be committed or forced to receive treatment in psychiatric hospitals. The second section, "Predicting Dangerousness", examines how reliably or accurately helping professionals are able to predict how dangerous people are.

The rights of patients in psychiatric facilities are covered in the third section of your text. You will discover that individuals in the United States have a right to either receive or refuse treatment. Your text then continues with an examination of insanity. Insanity is a legal, not psychological, concept. To say that someone is insane is to say that they are not legally responsible for their acts. Your text presents a brief history of the key legal cases that have led to the current controversy over insanity. There are two questions here that are still unresolved: Should insanity be a defense? And, under what conditions should we call someone insane? Although not a psychological concept, the opinion of helping professionals is often sought in making judgments about the sanity of an individual. Insanity is one of two legal principles under which persons may not be held responsible for their behavior under the law; incompetence is the other. A person must be found competent in order to stand trial. Following the topic on insanity, your text examines the principle of competence.

The last legal issue that your text examines is a helping professional's duty to warn third parties of potential danger from a client. This duty to warn has been established by two court cases, one from California and one from Vermont. Your text includes an extensive examination of the pros and cons of requiring therapists to warn others of the dangerousness of clients.

The chapter ends with an examination of two contemporary issues that confront helping professionals. The first is what to do about the large number of individuals who, because they are not dangerous, are being released from psychiatric hospitals even though they can in no way be considered "cured" of their abnormal behavior. You may find it amazing and disturbing to find that relatively little is being done for these persons. The second issue is how to prevent abnormal behavior from developing. Prevention is the primary focus of the emerging area of Community Psychology. Your text examines some of the methods used to provide primary, secondary, and tertiary prevention.

CHAPTER OUTLINE

Psychiatric Commitment
Predicting Dangerousness
    Problems in Predicting Dangerousness
        The Post-Hoc Problem
        The Problem in Leaping from the General to the Specific
        Problems in Defining Dangerousness
        Base Rate Problems
        The Unlikelihood of Disclosure of Direct Threats of Violence
        The Difficulty of Predicting Behavior in the Community from Behavior in
            the Hospital
Patient's Rights
    Right to Treatment
        O'Connor v. Donaldson
        Youngberg v. Romeo
    Right to Refuse Treatment
The Insanity Defense
    Legal Bases of the Insanity Defense
        Determining the Term of Criminal Commitment
        Perspectives on the Insanity Defense
Competency to Stand Trial
The Duty to Warn
        The Tarasoff Case
Preventing Psychological Disorders
    Primary Prevention
        "Soulbeat": A Sociocultural Perspective on Prevention
    Secondary Prevention
        Self Help Groups
        Telephone Hot Lines
        Community Consultation
        Early Intervention
    Tertiary Prevention
        Halfway Houses
    A Final Word on Prevention
Summary

LEARNING OBJECTIVES

The following learning objectives can also be found at the beginning of the chapter.
When you have completed your study of the chapter, you should be able to:

1.   Describe the legal procedures for psychiatric commitment.

2. Discuss the development of safeguards to prevent abuses of psychiatric commitment.
3. Discuss the controversy concerning psychiatric commitment.
4. Discuss research concerning the problems of psychologists and other professionals who are given the task of attempting to predict dangerousness.
5. Explain why professionals tend to overpredict dangerousness.
6. Discuss legal developments concerning the right to treatment.
7. Discuss legal developments concerning the right to refuse treatment.
8. Discuss the history of the legal bases of the insanity plea.
9. Discuss problems in determining the term of commitment for perpetrators who are found insane.
10. Discuss the problems that the insanity plea creates for jurors.
11. Discuss the guilty-but-mentally-ill verdict.
12. Discuss the issue of whether or not the insanity plea is degrading to the defendant.
13. Discuss the principle of competency to stand trial.
14. Explain the effects of the *Tarasoff* case on helping professionals' duty to warn third parties of threats posed by clients.
15. Discuss some of the conflicts involved in requiring helping professionals to warn third parties of threats.
16. Discuss the philosophy of prevention.
17. Discuss three kinds of prevention: primary, secondary, and tertiary.

KEY TERMS AND CONCEPTS

The following is a list of terms, concepts, and names that are discussed in the chapter. They are important for you to know. Review these terms, comparing your answers with the material presented in the text.

Civil/Psychiatric commitment
Legal commitment
Addington v. Texas
Thomas Szasz
Mental illness
Base-rate problem
False negative
False positive
Patient's rights
Wyatt v. Stickney
O'Connor v. Donaldson
Youngberg v. Romeo
Rogers v. Okin
Insanity defense
Insanity

Guilty-but-mentally-ill (GBMI) verdict
Durham v. United States
Mental disease/mental defect
ALI guideline
Jones v. United States
Jackson v. Indiana
Medina v. California
Tarasoff v. the Regents of the University of California
Duty to warn
Peck v. Counseling Service of Addison County
Primary prevention
Secondary prevention
Tertiary prevention
Health psychology
Systems-level strategy
Person-centered approach
Situation-focused approaches
Competence-enhancement approaches
Crisis intervention
Self-help groups
Telephone hot line
Community psychology
Early intervention
Halfway house

MATCHING

Match the following names, terms, and concepts with the definitions listed below. The answers are found at the end of the chapter.

a. tertiary prevention
b. false negative
c. Rogers v. Okin
d. primary prevention
e. insanity defense
f. crisis intervention
g. Wyatt v. Stickney
h. civil commitment
i. false positive
j. M'Naghten rule
k. health psychology
l. indeterminate commitment
m. Tarasoff v. Regents of the Univ. of California

n. community psychology
o. systems-level strategy
p. legal commitment
q. secondary prevention
r. Jackson v. Indiana
s. base-rate problem
t. Jones v. United States
u. Youngberg v. Romeo
v. voluntary hospitalization
w. ALI guideline
x. O'Connor v. Donaldson
y. competent to stand trial
z. Peck v. Counseling Services of Addison County

1) _____ may happen when a person is a threat to themselves or others

2) _____ requires therapists to reveal confidential information to protect property

3) _____ insane because one cannot tell right from wrong

4) _____ uncovering and eliminating the causes of abnormal behavior

5) _____ indeterminate commitment is legal for those not guilty through insanity

6) _____ allows a person to leave a psychiatric institution when they want

7) _____ a person who is capable of understanding criminal charges and proceedings

8) _____ no involuntary commitment for persons who are not dangerous

9) _____ focuses on changing society rather than changing the individual

10) _____ may happen when a person commits a crime due to a mental disorder or defect

11) _____ incorrectly failing to predict the occurrence of a behavior

12) _____ the field that focuses on using social systems to prevent and remedy abnormal behavior

13) _____ reducing the impact of abnormal behavior by providing rehabilitation

14) _____ combines the M'Naghten principle with the irresistible impulse principle

15) _____ a person cannot be confined longer than necessary to determine competency to stand trial

16) _____ the relative difficulty of making predictions of infrequent or rare events

17) _____ the claim of being not guilty due to a mental defect or disorder

18) _____ involves the coordination of emergency services to provide immediate help

19) _____ early intervention to prevent abnormal behavior from becoming severe

20) _____ psychotropic medications cannot be forced upon involuntarily committed patients

21) _____ treatment for the confined in reasonable safety

22) _____ when a person can be committed until their sanity is regained

23) _____ minimum standard of care for psychiatric hospitals

24) _____ incorrectly predicting the occurrence of a behavior

25) _____ the field that places a major emphasis on preventing physical illness by changing lifestyles

26) _____ requires therapists to reveal confidential information to protect third parties

TRUE-FALSE

The following true-false statements are reprinted here from your text. Can you remember the answers? They can be found at the end of this chapter.

1. _____ People can be psychiatrically committed because they are eccentric.
2. _____ Psychologists and psychiatrists can rely on their clinical judgment in making accurate predictions of the dangerousness of people they evaluate.
3. _____ An attempt to assassinate the president of the United States was seen by millions of television viewers, but the would-be assassin was found not guilty by a court of law.
4. _____ People who are found not guilty of a crime by reason of insanity may remain confined to a mental hospital indefinitely -- for many years longer than they would have been sentences to prison, if they had been found guilty.
5. _____ It is possible for a defendant to be held competent to stand trial but still be judged not guilty of a crime by reason of insanity.
6. _____ Therapists may not disclose confidential information about clients to third parties, even when their clients threaten violence to the third parties.

MULTIPLE CHOICE

The multiple choice questions listed below will test your understanding of the material presented in the chapter. Read through each question and circle the letter representing the best answer. The answers are found at the end of the chapter.

1) A psychologist tells a judge that a person should be hospitalized because they are a threat to themselves. If the judge agrees and hospitalizes the person, we have an example of what kind of commitment?

    a. civil commitment
    b. criminal commitment
    c. legal commitment
    d. voluntary commitment

2) In the GBMI (guilty but mentally ill) verdict, the defendant:

    a. is imprisoned
    b. can receive treatment
    c. may stay in prison longer because of the mental illness
    d. all of the above

3) Requiring therapists to warn third parties of threats by their clients may increase the risk of violence by their clients because:

    a. many violent people do not want to "look bad" by talking about it and not acting on it
    b. talking about the violent acts may make the person more apt to act on them
    c. therapists may be less willing to probe their clients about violent tendencies
    d. the client is very likely to direct the violence toward the therapist

4) In a study of homeless person in Los Angeles, _____ of the homeless had shown psychotic symptoms in the past two weeks.

    a. more than 80%
    b. about 40%
    c. about 10%
    d. less than 5%

5) Which of the following is an example of secondary prevention?

    a. suicide hot line
    b. halfway house
    c. communication skills training for engaged couples
    d. improved prenatal and perinatal care

6) Accuracy in predicting potential violence in a client is improved when it is based on:

    a. client self-report
    b. the client's behavior while hospitalized
    c. the client's past community behavior
    d. client self-report corroborated with reports from individuals who know the client well

7) What happens if a person is found incompetent to stand trial?

    a. they are found guilty but mentally ill and confined to a prison
    b. they are confined in a mental institution until they become competent
    c. they are immediately confined to a mental institution for life
    d. they are found not guilty by reason of insanity

8) Thomas Szasz believes that the insanity defense is degrading to defendants because it assumes that people:

    a. have free choice
    b. lack personal responsibility
    c. have personal determination
    d. are guilty until proven innocent

9) In Addington v. Texas, the United States Supreme Court ruled that a person can be involuntarily hospitalized:

    a. if they are "mentally ill" alone
    b. if they are a danger to themselves or others alone
    c. both of the above
    d. none of the above

10) The American Law Institute (ALI) guidelines to define insanity makes the decision of juries _____ because it _____ the number of cases in which the insanity plea could be used.

    a. harder; increases
    b. harder; decreases
    c. easier; increases
    d. easier; decreases

11) Which of the following must take place before an individual can be involuntarily placed in a psychiatric setting?

    a. a formal commitment petition must be filed with the court
    b. a complete psychiatric evaluation must be completed on the individual
    c. the individual must be currently engaged in treatment
    d. the individual must be deemed as a threat to themselves or others

12) One of the implications of the Tarasoff case is that:

    a. it ended the principle of therapist-client confidentiality
    b. it created the principle of therapist-client confidentiality
    c. it requires the therapists to breach therapist-client confidentiality
    d. it requires that clients assume the responsibility for asking therapists about the limits of confidentiality

13) Thomas Szasz has suggested which of the following?

    a. mental illness reflects an underlying medical problem
    b. people should not be deprived of their freedom simply because they appear different
    c. while the mental patient is dangerous society may also be dangerous
    d. mentally ill people who violate the law should go free because they are not responsible

14) The right to refuse treatment:

    a. has been established by the United States Supreme Court
    b. is legally recognized in about half of the United States
    c. has been legally recognized only in the state of Massachusetts
    d. has still not been legally recognized in the United States

15) Persons released from mental hospitals require:

    a. affordable housing
    b. alcohol abuse counseling
    c. social services
    d. all of the above

16) Which of the following is NOT an example of prevention?

    a. releasing psychiatric hospital patients
    b. stock piling grain in case of famine
    c. genetic counseling for newlyweds
    d. getting vaccinated against polio

17) All of the following are considered rights of the patient according to "The Patient's Bill of Rights under Wyatt v. Stickney" EXCEPT:

    a. nutritionally balanced diets
    b. suitable opportunities to interact with the opposite gender
    c. visitation and telephone privileges
    d. all of the above

18) In the case of Donaldson v. O'Connor, Kenneth Donaldson, the plaintiff in the case, was institutionalized by his father and:

    a. was provided with only occupational training while institutionalized
    b. refused medication while institutionalized
    c. was aggressively violent toward other members on his ward while institutionalized
    d. received no treatment whatsoever while institutionalized

19) Michael Jones was caught shoplifting, a crime with a maximum punishment of one year in prison. He was found not guilty by reason of insanity and:

    a. was released immediately
    b. was confined to a hospital for six months
    c. was confined to a hospital for one year
    d. was still confined to a hospital seven years after the crime occurred

20) The rights of patients to refuse psychotropic medications was tested in which of the following cases?

    a. Durham v. United States
    b. Rogers v. Okin
    c. Jones v. United States
    d. Medina v. California

21) Professionals overpredict violence in people with abnormal behavior because:

    a. they readily agree on what behavior is violent and dangerous
    b. behavior in hospital settings provide a good indicator for behavior in the community
    c. hospitalized individuals frequently issue specific threats to others
    d. violent acts in hospitals and society are relatively rare

22) Situation-focused and competence-enhancement approaches fall under which treatment approach?

   a. behavioral
   b. cognitive
   c. person-centered
   d. psychodynamic

23) "Soulbeat" is a culturally-specific substance abuse prevention program for which ethnic group?

   a. African Americans
   b. Mexican Americans
   c. Native Americans
   d. Asian Americans

24) Which of the following provides a structured living environment in the community for patients who do not require the more restrictive environment of an institution?

   a. intensive outpatient programs
   b. self-help facilities
   c. halfway houses
   d. crisis intervention support programs

25) The first insanity defense in history established that a person was not guilty because of:

   a. irresistible impulses due to a mental illness
   b. the inability to tell right from wrong
   c. the inability to understand the crime
   d. both a and c

QUESTIONS FOR CRITICAL THINKING

1.   Discuss why involuntary psychiatric commitment is controversial.
2.   Discuss the base-rate problem in predicting dangerousness.
3.   Discuss the implications of the Donaldson case to the field of psychology.
4.   Identify and discuss the hazards of patients refusing treatment.
5.   Discuss how the GBMI verdict has faired.
6.   Describe the insanity defense. Do you agree with this? Why or why not?
7.   Describe what makes the Durham rule unworkable.
8.   Discuss the implications of the Tarasoff decision for therapists. How might this impact therapy?

9.   Discuss how AIDS is related to the duty to warn. What are your personal thoughts about this dilemma?

10. Briefly describe the types of community programs available for psychiatric homeless.

11. Describe Soulbeat.

12. Discuss the role that halfway houses play in prevention.

13. Consider the following scenario: *Michael, an 18-year old male, was recently arrested for stealing. When he was picked up, he appeared to be hallucinating and expressed concern about someone trying to hurt him. While investigating the situation, it is discovered that Michael has been living with his mother who was diagnosed with paranoid schizophrenia when Michael was 3 years old. Since that time, they have been living in various homeless shelters and community parks. Michael was taken in and out of various school environments as a result of their homeless situation, and never graduated.* Now, discuss this case in terms of how primary, secondary, and tertiary prevention could be utilized to intervene in this situation.

ANSWERS FOR MATCHING

1.	h	10.	p	19.	q
2.	z	11.	b	20.	c
3.	j	12.	n	21.	u
4.	d	13.	a	22.	l
5.	t	14.	w	23.	g
6.	v	15.	r	24.	i
7.	y	16.	s	25.	k
8.	x	17.	e	26.	m
9.	o	18.	f		

TRUE-FALSE ANSWERS

1.	F	4.	T
2.	F	5.	T
3.	T	6.	F

MULTIPLE CHOICE ANSWERS

1.	a	11.	d	21.	d
2.	d	12.	c	22.	c
3.	c	13.	b	23.	a
4.	b	14.	b	24.	c
5.	a	15.	d	25.	b
6.	c	16.	a		
7.	b	17.	d		
8.	b	18.	d		
9.	c	19.	d		
10.	a	20.	b		